T0155143

CLUSTER HEADACHES
Treatment and Relief for Cluster, Cluster Migraine, and Recurring Eye-Stab Pain

By Michael Goldstein

New Atlantean Press
Santa Fe, New Mexico

CLUSTER HEADACHES
Treatment and Relief for Cluster, Cluster Migraine, and Recurring Eye-Stab Pain

By Michael Goldstein

International Standard Book Number:
1-881217-18-3
Library of Congress Catalog Card Number:
98-65663

Copyright © 1999 by Michael Goldstein

Cataloging-in-Publication Data
Goldstein, Michael (Michael E.) 1947-
    Cluster headaches : treatment and relief for cluster, cluster migraine, and recurring eye-stab pain / Michael Goldstein ; foreword by Seymour Diamond. -- 1st ed.
        p. cm.
    Includes index.   Preassigned LCCN: 98-65663
    1. Cluster headache--Treatment. 2. Migraine--Treatment.
    3. Eye-sockets--Diseases--Treatment. I. Title
RC392.G65 1999   616.8'491
ISBN: 1-881217-18-3 $9.95 softcover
                           QBI98-354

Printed in the United States of America

Published by:
New Atlantean Press
PO Box 9638-925
Santa Fe, NM 87504
Website: http://thinktwice.com/books.htm

TABLE OF CONTENTS

For additional information about cluster headaches, please visit:

http://clusterheadaches.com

This excellent site includes a cluster headache forum,
a live chat room, and other important cluster headache links.

*This book is dedicated to
cluster headache sufferers
and their families.*

Foreword

By Seymour Diamond, M.D.

As a headache clinician, the opportunity to review commentary provided by headache sufferers about their pain experiences and the various treatments offered has always been rewarding and insightful. The renditions provided in this text, by the cluster headache victims, are especially enlightening.

Cluster headache is not a common headache disorder, and like most pain problems it is difficult to objectively measure the degree of suffering. Only the cluster victim can understand the excruciating pain and discomfort that characterize this disorder. Fortunately, only a small percentage of cluster headache cases complain of the chronic form. Chronic cluster headache is distinguished by its lack of a remission period lasting more than 14 days, or the absence of a remission period for more than one year.

One of the earliest descriptions of the different forms of cluster headaches (episodic vs. chronic) was given by Bayard T. Horton, M.D. (1895-1980), of Mayo Clinic. Doctor Horton treated many of his chronic cluster headache patients with intravenous histamine desensitization. His work with this form of therapy was more or less abandoned during the last three decades. However, for those chronic cluster headache patients unresponsive to standard forms of therapy, the use of intravenous histamine desensitization may offer a viable alternative. At the Diamond Headache Clinic, this therapeutic modality is reserved for those chronic cluster headache patients refractory to all previous treatment options. It is my hope that by citing Doctor Horton's monumental work and his discernment about this debilitating condition, victims of chronic cluster headache will realize that other options are available to find relief.

The presentation of *this* book will also offer those with cluster headaches an insight into their condition, and a recognition that they are not alone in their suffering. The observations presented here will also be instructive for physicians managing similar cases.

Seymour Diamond, M.D.
Director, Diamond Headache Clinic
Director, Inpatient Headache Unit, Columbus Hospital
Chicago, Illinois

Introduction

Do you periodically experience excruciating pain behind one eye? Are medications relatively ineffective at providing relief? Is the pain so intense that you've thought about suicide? If so, then you may be suffering from cluster headaches, cluster migraines, or recurring eye-stab pain.

Although initially it was thought that only a small percentage of the population suffers from this debilitating condition, the numbers — about one in 400 — appear to be increasing. In fact, tens of thousands of men and women are directly or indirectly affected. Evidently, cluster victims are often misdiagnosed; many others suffer in silence, frustrated and embarrassed by their illness.

I am a cluster headache sufferer. For many years I have endured the agony of recurring eye-stab pain. Like many of my fellow sufferers, I desperately sought a respite from the unbearable ache, as well as the reason for this mysterious ailment. Today, although the cause continues to remain an enigma, new treatments offer better options for relief.

This book contains excerpts from the personal experiences of 217 cluster headache victims (and a few of their doctors). Each individual told his or her story in their own words. No questionnaire was provided.

The information in this book is provided to encourage and support cluster victims, their families, and the doctors who are trying to help. The comments in each chapter represent typical remarks. Statistical data is included in the appendix.

It is my sincere hope that a cause and cure for cluster headaches will soon be discovered. In the meantime, some clues about this condition, and promising methods to treat and relieve the pain, are included in the pages to follow. Good luck in your quest for a happy and healthy life.

Michael E. Goldstein
Chief Medical Researcher, NAP

Symptoms

The telltale signs of a cluster headache are distinct, as well as remarkably similar among cluster sufferers everywhere. Here is a list of commonly reported symptoms associated with this condition: a piercing, stabbing pain on one side of the head and behind the eye; the attacks occur in clusters lasting several weeks, with a remission period of months or years between headache cycles; several headaches daily, recurring at the same time each day, often awakening one from sleep; the inability to lay down or remain still; the eye becomes droopy, red and moist; the nostril on the affected side becomes stuffed and runny; the desire to pound one's head against the wall; dejection, anxiety, and irritability.

Comments:

[1055] A cluster headache is an excruciating vascular headache. It is similar to migraine, but shorter in duration, more frequently occurring, and more severe. It affects men more than women, and is much more rare than migraine. A cluster headache usually begins around or behind the eye. It may spread to the temple, jaw, cheek, neck, and back of head. Attacks arrive in clusters, lasting weeks to months, with months or years between headache cycles. Sometimes cluster headaches become chronic, in which case they do not go into a remission. The actual headache lasts from 30 minutes up to two hours. This may happen once a day or multiple times daily.

[1066] A typical symptom of mine is the inability to stay still due to the unbearable pain.

[1087] My clusters are always on my right side, behind my eye. I can't keep my eye open at the peak. It becomes watery and red. I feel like pounding my head on a wall.

[1088] In the early years, pain began in my shoulder blade and then crept up into my head. Once in my head, I would experience, in addition to the classic pain behind my right eye, intermittent but frequent bursts of pain in other areas on the right side of my head.

[1093] My clusters are normally only on one side of the head. They usually commence 30 minutes to one-and-a-half hours after I lay down for the evening. My eye will get very red and will tear up uncontrollably (the other eye remains clear). The most intense pain is located over the eye and sometimes gravitates to the temple area, then around the ear to the lower back portion of the skull. I seldom get a cluster during the day, and I experience a minimum of two, and up to five, every night during the peak cycle. Also, during the headaches, I am light and sound sensitive.

[1095-F] My clusters always come at night after I just lay down. I have to get up because the pain is so intense, and laying down seems to make it worse. I cannot seem to sit still during a cluster; I either pace, rock my body back and forth, or pound my head.

[1101] Clusters cause brutal pain to my left eye and to the left side of my face, a droopy left eye, and nasal stoppage.

[1109] I experience tearing of the eye, pressure behind the eye, drooping of the eyelid, intense pain, and light sensitivity. I can't lie down when I'm in the middle of an attack because the pain becomes even more severe. I have also experienced some nausea.

[1124] I suffer from cluster headaches behind my right eyeball and around to the back of my head, always in the right hemisphere. They strike at the same time every day for two weeks or more.

[1127-F] My headaches are always on the same side. My eye on the affected side tears and my nostril on the same side becomes "stopped up." I can't lay down when I have an attack, although moving around does not make the pain go away. I sometimes feel nauseous. They wake me from sleep, but there is no indication that I am going to get a headache before I retire for the evening.

[1145-F] The most classic symptom is waking up in the middle of the night with intense pain. It is so bad that you may end up in the hospital. The pain is worse lying down, so you end up pacing.

[1151] The pain is always on my right side, behind the eye.

[1158-F] Cluster headaches come in clusters then go into remission (except chronic sufferers who experience no periods of remission).

[1161] My clusters wake me after I am sound asleep. A burning sensation occurs high up in my sinus cavity, like an ice pick behind my right eye. I get the impression that I have some raging infection eating my head out from the inside. My eye is bloodshot and tears. I get up, pace, and try to keep myself from crying and screaming. I try to keep calm but I have a tremendous desire to thrash about. Thrashing does not help, nor does yelling or head banging. I hold my right temple and almost go crazy. I can't compose myself or communicate with others. When it goes away, I fall into bed and crash. Unfortunately, 45 minutes or so later the whole process repeats itself. This occurs another three to four times a night. By morning I am a wreck. My head is tender and sore to the touch, and I feel dull for the rest of the day.

[1162] I get warning symptoms when the cycle is about to begin. It's hard to explain how I know they are about to start. I am afraid to go to sleep at night. When the precursor pain wakes me, I know that I must immediately get out of bed to begin countermeasures. After several days of this, I find that I try to stay in bed and just let it come hoping the cycle will finish and I can get back to normal. Of course, once the pain gets started it is impossible to remain still.

[1163-F] They are always on the right side of my face, along my nose, up into my temple, and sometimes far up into my scalp. It feels like a vise is clamping down on my face. My face and neck swell before a cycle starts.

[1164] Cluster headaches are unusually severe headaches that occur in bunches, or "clusters." They last from a few minutes to a few hours. In between these clusters of headaches the patient can go for long periods — weeks, months, or even years — without an attack. Once a cluster period begins, headache frequency varies depending on the individual. Severe head pain can occur several times a day, week, or month. Cluster headaches usually worsen over time, reach a peak of frequency, duration, and severity, and then generally diminish or disappear after age 40. Unfortunately, not everyone follows this pattern, and there are cluster sufferers in their late 60s.

[1171] A cluster is different than a migraine. A cluster sufferer is a screamer and a head banger.

[1174] Cluster headaches begin as pain around one eye, eventually spreading to that side of the face. The pain quickly intensifies, compelling the victim to pace the floor. Other symptoms include a stuffed and runny nose and a droopy eyelid over a red and tearing eye. Cluster headaches may last between 30 and 45 minutes, but the relief people feel at the end of an attack is usually mixed with dread as they await a recurrence. Clusters can strike several times a day for several weeks or months. Then, they may disappear for months or years. Many people get them during the spring and fall. Chronic cluster headaches can last continuously for years. Cluster attacks can strike at any age but often start between the ages of 20 and 40.

[1175] Symptoms begin with an odd sensation, similar to sinus pressure, on the left side of my head. The roof of my mouth on the left side begins to ache. Next, the whole left side of my head,

9

including the large vein running along the side of my head, the top of my head, eye, ear, and jaw become red and painful. My eye will swell, tear, and turn red. My nose will run as well. The severe pain radiates down the back of my skull and into my neck. Sometimes I feel as though I become disoriented and slow. I become agitated and restless for the duration of the attack.

[1181] My eye tears, my nostril becomes stuffy, and I experience excruciating pain on the right side of my head, especially in and around my eye. The pain moves down into my neck.

[1195] Cluster episodes can skip years, but expect the frequency of headaches to increase as you age. During the worst pain, I may experience a temporary loss of vision in my left eye.

[1204] I walk back and forth in a darkened room, counting each trip to occupy my mind. I used to pound my head against the wall, but my head would be so sore the next day that I stopped.

[1219-F] Sometimes my speech slurs, I can't think clearly, I get nauseated, and feel that I'm having an out-of-body experience.

[1222] I have problems with speech during the cycle.

[1224] During an attack I become irritable and feel terribly alone. I can't sit still; I'm constantly rubbing my hair and eyes, blowing my nose, and clenching my teeth.

[1238-F] I am unable to remain still during an attack. There is sinus congestion, as well as pain and pressure behind the eye.

[1242] Cluster headaches are characterized by sudden, intense, unilateral head pain, usually centering around the eye. Attacks often occur one to three hours after going to sleep (during rapid eye movement — REM), and last about an hour. Cluster headaches tend to recur night after night for weeks or months, then disappear for months or years. Some patients experience as many as eight to ten headaches during a 24 hour period.

[1246] Cluster headaches only occur during a cluster period.

[1258] I experience a piercing, stabbing pain behind my left eye or between my eye and temple area. I have gone for months without them, then wham, it shows up again and will last for weeks.

[1265-F] I get a few seconds "notice" before a cluster starts.

Initial Diagnosis

General consensus indicates that most doctors are unfamiliar with the specific disorder known as *cluster headache*. More often than not, it isn't even a diagnostic option to the health practitioner. Therefore, even though the patient may display many or all of the classic cluster symptoms, a misdiagnosis is highly probable.

Many cluster sufferers report that they have been to numerous doctors, neurologists and other specialists, over a period of years, prior to being accurately diagnosed. In addition to their pain, they have incurred great frustration in seeking answers to their little known condition, untold expense, and have been subjected to a number of inappropriate treatments.

Here is a partial list of conditions erroneously attributed to the cluster sufferer. They are presented in an approximate order of their misdiagnosis: The ailment is a mystery; migraine (most often ascribed to female sufferers); sinus complications; allergies; stress and physical tension; eye strain (or the need for a new eyeglass prescription); brain tumors (or the need for an MRI, CAT scan, and x-rays); psychological causes; vascular headaches; impacted teeth; a deviated septum.

Comments:

[1051] The many doctors that I saw weren't sure what my problem was. I went from one doctor to another, trying different things. Nothing helped. When I was finally diagnosed with clusters, the doctors I saw were relatively new to this problem. The neurologists I saw knew of clusters but related them to migraines.

[1066] I was told by general practitioners and specialists that I was suffering from migraine headaches. When I found a neurologist it become clear that I am suffering from "Horton's headache."

[1069] I went to a number of doctors, over a seven year period, who didn't have a clue. I took histamine shots, psychotherapy, and ineffective drugs. Find a good neurologist.

[1075] At first, I thought there was a problem with my contacts because the pain always started in my left eye. My doctor didn't know what they were because by the time I got to his office they would be gone.

[1081] My husband has been to numerous doctors, had surgery to correct a deviated septum, CAT scans, x-rays, and has tried just about anything that anyone would prescribe.

[1087] I really feel for those who are just starting to get them in their teens, like I did at the age of 15. The pain they will have to go through, and the frustration they will experience in trying to find a doctor who will understand, makes me angry.

[1088] In the early years, my clusters seemed to be correlated with stress, so I assumed they were tension headaches.

[1092] I've had clusters for about ten years, but did not know what I had until five years ago.

[1111] The doctors said it was an allergy, and sent me to a specialist who agreed with him. The allergist tested me and said I was allergic to dust, mites that live on the dust, grass, and pollen. In short, I was allergic to life! He said that the pain was because of the reaction to this, and I would need to come in and get two shots twice a week. Trying to get rid of the pain, I went for two years. After the second year I started to talk to some of the other patients and discovered that we were all, in fact, allergic to everything — even though we weren't there for the same reasons. I went back to my family doctor and asked him to get me some help. Finally, he contacted a head pain clinic. The neurologist diagnosed me with cluster headaches. What a relief. Now what to do!

[1120] I was misdiagnosed with everything from migraine, to stress headaches, to trigeminal neuralgia.

[1130] I was diagnosed as having severe sinus problems that could only be fixed by surgery. Not knowing anything about headaches at the time, I had the surgery, and the ear, nose, and throat doctor (ENT) made his money. I was back six months later with another episode of headaches. I thought he had screwed up the surgery. Then I read an article on cluster headaches, got another opinion, and started dealing with it.

[1132] My headaches were first diagnosed as "sinus," and when the medicine didn't work, the doctor said "cluster."

[1140] After going to two pain and headache clinics at a cost of three thousand dollars each, my condition was finally diagnosed as cluster headaches with migraine components.

[1141] I've suffered from cluster headaches for 16 years, only knowing what they were for the past six years. Before I was correctly diagnosed, I had been to allergists, chiropractors, and doctors who were sure I had sinus infections. I finally saw a neurologist and started getting some proper treatment.

[1144] The doctor gave me a blood test, an MRI, and a CAT scan. His diagnoses was "vascular" headache. He sent me home with the headache still intact.

[1145-F] My doctor was supposed to be a top neurologist. He misdiagnosed my headaches as migraines.

[1158-F] I went from doctor to doctor trying to find out what was wrong with me. Each one said "migraine," and put me on migraine medication. That was not the solution. I searched on my own until I discovered that my ailment was "cluster headaches." My next battle was to convince the doctor that was what I needed treatment for.

[1159] I have suffered from clusters for 19 years, but it was only three years ago that a neurologist correctly diagnosed my condition.

[1164] I find it interesting that doctors often diagnose women with something other than cluster headache, even when the symptoms are obvious, the reason being that "women don't get clusters."

[1165] I found out what I had this year, not because my doctors told me, but through all of the reading I've done.

[1166] During my first episode, the doctor arranged for me to have a CAT scan. During my next episode, the new doctors found that my right eye was weaker than my left, so they gave me a prescription for glasses. When the clusters returned, I went to a neurologist. Even he didn't know what I had, or how to treat them. My wife called a headache clinic and they correctly diagnosed clusters.

[1167] I went from Dr. A to Dr. B, who sent me to Dr. C, who recommended me to Dr. A. Finally, a neurologist diagnosed me with Horton's syndrome.

[1189-F] When I go to the emergency room with a cluster headache, the doctor's don't believe me because I am 25, female, don't smoke or drink, and am at a normal weight. But, the pain that I experience is definitely not a migraine.

[1197] At first my doctor tested me for allergies.

[1199] Years ago I was told that they were vascular headaches.

[1203] I went through the typical runaround at first, from doctor to doctor, until I was correctly diagnosed.

[1205-F] Because I am a female, the medical profession constantly tried to diagnose me with migraines, but finally diagnosed cluster.

[1207] No doctor was able to diagnose what was wrong with me. I visited a neurologist, eye doctor, back doctor, and several more to no avail. Eventually I found a medical book that accurately described the symptoms and called the disease "Horton's headache."

[1218-F] About 20 years ago I noticed that some "migraines" were much worse than others, and were accompanied by one-sided congestion, one eye swelling and drooping with tears, with the pupil constricted on that side. One doctor diagnosed me with clusters, but others have been skeptical since I am female. My current doctor thinks it doesn't help to differentiate between clusters and regular migraines because "they're all on a continuum of headaches." It matters to me because the clusters are a lot more intense. He doesn't realize how much worse the clusters are.

[1219-F] My head pains were always diagnosed as sinus headaches. Finally, a doctor told me that I had clusters. It is hard to convince other doctors that what I have is not a sinus infection.

[1224] During my initial bout, I went to three different doctors for diagnosis. They suspected everything from eye-strain, sinus infection, and ear infection, to smelly feet and nasty disposition. When this first episode subsided, I figured that it was indeed some sort of an infection that resolved itself. Four years later, during my next attack, a couple of new doctors did some more guessing. Then my brother-in-law, a doctor, figured it out.

[1249] It was only this year, after five years of suffering, that I found out what was wrong. My doctor said I had sinus problems. I went to an ear, nose, and throat specialist for help with my "sinus." He wanted to operate. My wife began doing research and found that I have cluster headaches. My doctor ultimately agreed. From what I've read, "sinus" is a common misdiagnosis.

[1251] I was misdiagnosed for seven years before getting referred to a neurologist.

[1257] I've had my nose broken by the ear, nose, and throat guys, my wisdom teeth pulled by the TMJ guys, and been given every pain medicine in the book before I was properly diagnosed.

Onset and Duration

In this chapter, cluster headache sufferers offer details about their current age, their age at the onset of the initial symptoms, and the number of years they have suffered from cluster headaches. A complete analysis of this data may be found in the appendix on page 73. Some general observations are noted below:

More than half (52 percent) of all cluster sufferers in this study were under the age of 40. Just 15 percent were at least 50 years old. Eighty-four percent were under the age of 30 when their symptoms began, and nearly half (47 percent) were under the age of 20 when their headaches started. In fact, the average age of female sufferers at the time of onset was 18 years. Only four percent of all sufferers were at least 40 years old when their cycles began. The average victim has suffered for at least 15 years, but only nine percent has had to endure clusters for more than 25 years.

Comments:

[1051] I'm a 46 year old professional male who was diagnosed a little over nine years ago with cluster headaches.

[1052] I have suffered from cluster headaches for more than 25 years — ever since I was 27 years old. I am 54 years old now.

[1053] I am 45 years old, and have been living with cluster headaches for about 25 years now.

[1054] My husband has been suffering from clusters since he was 17 years old. He is now 30 years old.

[1061] I am now 23 years old and have been experiencing cluster headaches since I was 18 years old.

[1063] I am 38 years old and have led a healthy active life. I have suffered from cluster headaches since I was 18 years old.

[1068-F] My 37 year old wife has suffered from cluster headaches for the past 16 years, starting when she was 21 years old.

[1075] I am only 18 years old, but have been getting cluster headaches for three years.

[1077] I'm a 36 year old male, and I have been suffering with cluster headaches for the past 18 years.

[1086] I am 34 years old and have suffered from cluster headaches since the age of fourteen.

[1087] I am 32 years old and have been having clusters for more than 16 years, since I was about 15 years old.

[1094-F] I am a 40 year old female, and have had cluster headaches since I was 16 years old.

[1095-F] I have suffered for the past seven years from what the doctors call "chronic" cluster headaches.

[1096] I am 35 years old, and have had clusters since I was 16 years old.

[1097] I am a 50 years old. My clusters started four years ago.

[1099] I'm 36 years old, and have suffered from cluster headaches for 18 years.

[1104] I have suffered from cluster headaches for 25 years, ever since I was 14 years old.

[1111] My clusters started 12 years ago, when I was 26 years old.

[1114] I am a 45 year old welder. I started suffering from cluster headaches about three years ago.

[1116] My husband is 42 years old. He has suffered with clusters since the third grade. I met a teacher in the neurology office the other day who has a second grader with clusters.

[1121] I'm a 32 year old male who has suffered from cluster headaches for nearly 15 years now.

[1128] I have suffered from cluster headaches for 25 years. I first started getting them when I was 17 years old.

[1130] I started getting cluster headaches in college, 12 years ago.

[1136] I'm 46 years old and have had these clusters for 20 years.

[1143] I have experienced cluster headaches since I was about ten years old. I am now 52 years old.

[1145-F] I started getting clusters at the age of 14. I'm 49 now.

[1146-F] I started getting these nightmare headaches in my teens.

[1153] I am 26 years old and have been suffering from chronic clusters since I was 18.

[1154] I've had clusters for the past 15 years, since I was 25.

[1156-F] I have had clusters since I was 16. I am 34 years old.

[1157] I'm now going on 69 years. I've had clusters for over 40 years, since I was diagnosed in my 20s.

[1158-F] My clusters started when I was 16. I'm now 33.

[1159] I've had clusters for 20 years now. I'm a 37 year old male.

[1166] I've been getting these headaches now for over 15 years. I started getting them when I was 25. My uncle started getting his in his 30s. He is 70 now, and hasn't had them since he was in his 50s.

[1171] I am a chronic cluster sufferer for almost 20 years now.

[1174] I've had cluster migraines for six years. I'm a 31 years old.

[1175] I have suffered from classic cluster migraine headaches for the past 15 years.

[1179] I've had to endure three clusters over the last four years. I'm 23 years old.

[1181] I am a 40 year old male. I started having cluster headaches when I was 19 years old.

[1191] I'm 39 year old male. I've been suffering from cluster headaches for at least 25 years now.

[1193] I've suffered from this god-forsaken illness for 12 years.

[1195] I've had cluster headaches since I was 17. I am now 43.

[1197] I started getting clusters when I was 27. I am now 35.

[1199] I've suffered since age 16 and am now 35.

[1204] My first cluster appeared when I was 35. I am now 51.

[1207] I'm a 31 year old male who has suffered from cluster headaches since around ten years old.

[1209] I am a 41 year old male and have suffered from clusters on and off since 1977.

[1211-F] I have suffered form cluster and migraine headaches since my mid twenties. I am 46 now.

[1213] I've been having cluster headaches for 16 years now, half my life.

[1216] I am a 50 year old male who has been suffering from cluster headaches for about 20 years.

[1218-F] I was in my 20s when my clusters began.

[1219-F] I am a 28 year old female and I found out I had clusters when I was 17.

[1224] I am a 61 year old married male who has suffered on and off for about 15 years.

[1228-F] I am a female, 50, who has suffered from clusters since my middle 20s.

[1232] I've suffered from cluster headaches since High School.

[1238-F] I have been having cluster headaches since I was eight years old. I am now 32.

[1249] I'm 35 years old and have been suffering from clusters for the past five years.

[1255] I started my cluster headaches 27 years ago at the age of 25.

[1261] I was diagnosed with cluster headaches at 21, and have suffered for over 15 years.

[1263-F] I am a 19 year old cluster sufferer.

[1264-F] I am 31 years old and have been suffering for six years.

[1265-F] I have had clusters since I was 20; I am now 29 years old.

[1266] I am 50 years old and have suffered since my early 20s.

Recurring Cycles

Cluster cycles appear to exist among individual sufferers, as well as within the group as a whole. But the recurring patterns are imprecise and variable. They are subject to change from event to event in frequency, duration, and pain intensity. For example, many respondents report that for many years the span of time between episodes was consistent, then mysteriously changed. Or that episodes always ended after a certain number of weeks...except that the current episode broke the pattern. Or that the attacks always occur in the evening and last for a certain number of hours...except that now they've shifted to mornings and the pain is more severe. A complete summary of recurring cluster cycles is included in the appendix on page 74.

<u>Comments</u>:

[1050] They occur every couple of years, lasting from one to three months. I have heard that they tend to go away with age. I am 63 years old now, and have been free of them for about five years, so maybe I am out of the woods.

[1051] I get hit every three to four years with episodes lasting about three months. I am presently in a session that is going on four months. I am near the end of this session because that is when the headaches become very, very intense! As most cluster sufferers know, what appears to work during a previous episode doesn't work for another. It appears that the "nature" of cluster headaches changes from episode to episode.

[1052] I have had clusters start at any time of year. My episodes were fairly short in the beginning, lasting a couple of weeks about every year. Then they changed to every two years, but the duration seemed to get longer each time until I had a cluster period of about five months. That was when I was 44 years old. Since then, the time between cluster episodes has increased to about every three years and the durations are now about three months. I have read that one will eventually outgrow clusters. I sure hope it is soon.

[1053] My clusters have never gone away, although sometimes they diminish in intensity and frequency.

[1055] My clusters never stop — from two to five attacks a day — except once they gave me a three or four week respite.

[1057] Every 22 to 23 months I can count on a period of two to three months of hell. I've identified three stages to my cluster attacks, which I call Early, Peak, and Waning. In the Early period, at the start of a cycle, the first attack is subtle — a very short stab of pain in the left temple area. The next day, at more or less the same time, it hits again. This will continue for a number of weeks during which time the pain intensity increases as does the duration and number of attacks per day. During the Peak period all hell breaks loose. Attacks are now three per day at irregular intervals. One of the three attacks is so excruciating that I have not yet found any medication to deal with it. Peak period attacks last two to three weeks. During the Waning period the cluster loses its intensity and frequency until it disappears for 22 to 23 months.

[1061] I get cluster headaches every fall around the end of October. During the first week, I get one about every other day. As time goes on they become more frequent and much, much more intense.

[1066] My clusters come in intervals, two periods per year. During peak periods, I experience five to six attacks per day.

[1067] My husband suffers from cluster headaches every four years for two months at a time.

[1068-F] Seven years ago my cluster headaches became chronic. One season lasted 11 months.

[1069] My clusters occur in 12 to 18 month cycles, from December through April and August through October. They occur about four to seven times per day, mostly at night.

[1070] I get clusters every 18 to 24 months for about three months at a time.

[1071] I have had cluster headaches several times a day, almost every day, for 25 years.

[1072] I've had clusters two or three times a year for the first ten years. Each time it took longer to disappear. Last year's cluster "visited" me for four months, with two to four attacks per day.

[1073] I have suffered from clusters in four to five year cycles.

[1075] I get clusters almost exactly when spring arrives. I only have them for about three weeks, but I get them every day during that time, and they start at the same time everyday. Somehow I didn't get them this spring, but I am scared I will get them again.

[1077] My cluster cycles are usually in the winter months, from late December through April, although on rare occasions I have had a cycle in the late summer months.

[1079-F] Every year, around April or May, my 40 year old sister experiences six or seven weeks of daily cluster headaches.

[1081] My husband has gone for as long as one year without a cluster headache. His cycles generally last two to three months, with one headache per day, usually at night.

[1082] My clusters are spaced about a year to a year-and-a-half apart, lasting two months. I get ten or twelve headaches per day.

[1086] I am currently in the 16th day of a cluster period — not the longest but definitely the most severe period that I have had since about the age of 23. This particular cluster is occurring after nearly seven years of no significant cluster period.

[1087] My clusters are absent for 12 to 18 months, then the episodes last for a month to six weeks with two to ten headaches a day. I'm praying for an end soon.

[1088] My most recent attack only abated after ten months. They have been under control but have not gone away entirely.

[1090] I'm having what seems to be a precursor to the return of my cluster headaches. These are small headaches occurring on the left side rather than on the right where they have always been.

[1091] I get clusters three to six months a year. The worst ever was nine months. It went from the left side to the right side. My clusters occur every two to three hours and last about one-and-a-half hours.

[1095] I am a chronic sufferer, which means that I get hit with one to two unbearable cluster headaches once a week — usually on the same day and at the same time.

[1103] My clusters are on the left side and last up to six months.

[1109] I'm currently in the 18th day of this cycle after a 23 month respite. My cycles typically last for two-and-a-half to three months — so I haven't hit the really desperate phase yet.

[1112] My husband has been suffering from multiple, daily cluster headaches for the past nine months.

[1114] My headaches come during the winter, usually lasting from October to February.

[1118] My clusters came every couple of years until I broke out of that pattern. Now I have chronic cluster and migraine headaches. I am presently having two to three headaches every day.

[1121] Without exception, I get my headaches every year in the fall, from September through late November. During this period I get them every day, sometimes several times per day. They last anywhere from one-and-a-half to four hours. When they are short, I can usually expect others during the day.

[1123] My cluster cycles last for up to six months. Recently they have started up again after only a three week headache-free period.

[1126] I am one of the very few people whose cluster headaches went chronic. Now there is very little relief. I have them all the time; sometimes they are easy to keep under control, and other times, like during July and August, they have been a real bear.

[1127] Originally, the headaches started about half an hour after I went to sleep. I would wake with a severe pain on the right side of my head. During the last cycle I was awake when 90 percent of the headaches started. The cycles I have now last about four to five weeks, with a headache every other day.

[1128] For the first twelve years my cluster cycles would come every spring or summer. I would get them for three months, every other day at ten in the morning, like clockwork. They would last for one hour and then stop. They always occurred on the left side of my head. During the last twelve years they switched. Instead of the "season" lasting three months, it now lasts about three weeks. But they are more frequent and intense. Now, instead of getting them every other day at ten in the morning, I get them every night at ten in the evening, and sometimes five to six per night, each one lasting a half hour or so. And they moved to the right side of my head. I've had only four hours of sleep in the last three days. As soon as I try to sleep it nails me again, and this lasts all night.

[1132] They hit like clockwork two hours after going to sleep.

[1136] My last rest was for 18 months. Wow, what a break. I thought I was over them but I'm in a cycle now which started in November. I'm getting four or five headaches a day.

[1145-F] My episodes are typically every three years lasting for a month. This time, I'm getting an episode after only two years.

[1149] Mine quit being clusters and turned to the chronic form.

[1150] I get as many as five headaches a week. I used to have long stretches of time without headaches, but the headache-free periods seem to be diminishing.

[1151] My episodes last about three weeks, twice a year. I get them every day at 8:30 in the morning and 7:30 in the evening.

[1152] I had episodic clusters for nine years; they converted to chronic two years ago.

[1154] My clusters come in the spring and fall. During episodes, my headaches always come one to two hours after I fall asleep, and are always on the right side of my head near my temple.

[1156-F] I am a rare woman cluster sufferer. Every August I just try to survive this six to eight week period.

[1157] I have had clusters since the 1950s. My cluster frequency and severity has varied dramatically. Some of my cycles lasted three to four months; others only ten days or so. I think I might have "outgrown" mine. I've had none for almost two years now. My previous longest interval between cycles was about 18 months.

[1159] For about 12 years my clusters stayed at about the same frequency and intensity: one cycle per year for about four to five weeks, usually one per day, lasting an hour. Then in 1989 they started getting worse — lasting up to four hours. However, the good news is that since 1991 the cycles are getting further apart.

[1160] My cycles fluctuate; some have lasted two months and others have lasted six months.

[1161] Getting older has its benefits. The remission period between clusters seems to increase. My recent "vacation" from the clusters has lasted over three years. I am now in the 3rd week of my new cycle. Hopefully, I have only a few more weeks to go. They don't last more than two months. Most of my headaches occur at night, usually after a couple of hours of sound sleep. They get worse as the night progresses. I get from three to six per evening, but after awhile they start to slide over into the day. Each attack lasts 30 to 35 minutes. I actually watch the clock, waiting for it to be over.

[1162] My cycle is changing as I grow older. During my 20s I had a cycle every other year that would last for about six weeks, with each session lasting about one hour. My early 30s saw a cycle once a year. The cycle still lasted six weeks, but each session was longer, up to two hours. In the last six years I've only had two cycles. I hope this is sign that the cluster monster is going away.

[1163-F] It visits me every three years and lasts for ten weeks. But last time it came after only one year. They happen once a night or they wake me, and they last from 45 minutes to four hours.

[1166] I get my headaches in the spring and the fall like clockwork. They usually last from one-and-a-half to two months, with each headache waking me up an hour after I fall asleep.

[1171] I am chronic, and never without clusters, but I do go through times when I only get several a week instead of every day. Mine last between two-and-a-half and three hours.

[1174] I am a chronic cluster sufferer. I have gone at most for a month or two without headaches.

[1181] My headaches usually last two and a half months. Last year they began in October and lasted six months.

[1182] I haven't noticed anything seasonal because I am a chronic sufferer; my clusters are year round.

[1187-F] I have between two and 17 cluster headaches per week.

[1191] My cluster cycle occurs only on odd years (1991, 1993, 1995, etc.) They may also be seasonal, starting in early October and lasting between six to ten weeks. They usually occur once a day during this period.

[1193] My clusters usually last six to eight weeks, and only skipped a year one time. The cycle that I am in now is different than years past. Before, my headaches were like clockwork occurring between 3 o'clock and 5 o'clock in the morning. With this cluster, I've been getting up to four headaches a day at different times.

[1195] When I was in my twenties, two years would pass between episodes. In my early thirties, one year. In my late thirties, months. I am now seldom without them. My pain cycles average nine days and range from three to 14 days or more. Off-periods (no headache) last two or three days before it begins again.

[1196] The first year was the worst. The headache lasted nearly four months. They generally last about six weeks now, and can start anytime between March and April.

[1198] The cycles used to occur every 18 months. We could set our calendars to it! They lasted for two weeks, then they would be gone for another 18 months. During the two week episode, my husband would have from one to ten headaches a day.

[1204] I can set my clock with the onset of the headaches. Right now, they show up at 2:30 in the afternoon and 10:15 in the evening. They begin as a tightness in my neck, and gradually build. I have about 30 minutes to find a place to suffer. They last from one to two hours. The cycles generally end with an all-night episode.

[1206] My clusters used to occur every three or four years, lasting anywhere from four to six weeks at a time. Sometimes they hit in the early spring, sometimes in the middle of winter, but they only struck once a year. In the last two years, my frequency has changed; I now have two "seasons" of headaches every year!

[1209] In the past I have gone anywhere from six months to 18 months between clusters. They usually occur in the fall and spring. It has been two years since my last bout, but they always seem to come back. I am currently in another session of clusters that started January 1997. This year I seem to be a little early. I do, however, believe this bout has been less intense than previous ones.

[1212] I've gotten better at aborting a cluster attack, but this just seems to store it up for a bigger one later on. At first, my attacks were exclusively at the onset of REM sleep in the first 90 minute sleep cycle of each night, with no recurrences during the same night. But this time, probably due to a European trip I took before the start of the episode, the attacks are at any time of day, mainly in the early evening.

[1216] I keep waiting to outgrow them but I find that I am, once again, in cycle.

[1217] My particular brand strikes between three and four in the morning, first every day, and now every other day.

[1218-F] The headaches become more frequent as I get older.

[1222] I had a cycle of clusters last August that lasted about two months. It had been 22 months since I had a cycle before that. I get my headaches about one hour after falling asleep. The cluster pain lasts one to two hours with some of headaches lasting over three hours. Once my cluster are in full bloom I will receive multiple headaches each evening and I start going to bed later each night. I live on two hours of sleep each evening for about six weeks.

[1223] My current cluster cycle has lasted 11 months. Prior to this one, my longest cycle was three months. My neurologist says that they become chronic in some people. I hope to god he's wrong.

[1224] The first series of cluster attacks came about 15 years ago and lasted for two weeks. The next series of attacks came four years later. The pain lasted one week. The third series of attacks didn't occur again for five years. Attacks lasted anywhere from half an hour to an hour. Each episode in this latest bout that I am going through lasts anywhere from one to four hours.

[1226] Every two years I would go through a series of attacks lasting six months. In 1994 they became chronic until December 1996.

[1228] My clusters occur every two years and last for five weeks. They can come during any season. My clusters primarily wake me from sleep, although I do get some during the day while awake. I have had as many as six episodes of pain a night.

[1249] My bouts start anytime between December and April, last about four months, and get worse as they progress. I just ended a five month bout this past August. That was the longest one yet.

[1255] When my clusters first started, the pain would last a short time, probably 15 to 30 minutes. The headaches would strike at random and did not seem to come in the clusters that they later developed into. As the years have gone by, the clusters have grown further apart — sometimes as much as a year. However, the pain has become more intense and lasts longer, sometimes four to eight hours. I just had a cluster that started in January and lasted for one month. During a cluster, the headaches "repeat" at intervals of 24, 36, 48 or 72 hours. Once a pattern is established for that cluster, the headaches seem to follow closely. This recent cluster occurred 24 months after the previous one — the longest time ever between clusters. I really thought that they might be over, but not so.

[1265-F] The pain increases from headache to headache during the cycle. I used to get them once every two years, then once a year. There was only a six month gap between the last two episodes.

Pain

Cluster victims are compelled to experience a considerable degree of suffering. Many gain a small measure of comfort in knowing that other people realize the true extent of their agonizing affliction. Here is a list of expressions frequently used by cluster sufferers to describe their pain: hard to comprehend; impossible to describe; like an ice pick stuck in my eye; like a knife plunged through my temple; excruciating; unbearable; suicidal; devastating; severe; intense; fierce; brutal; torturous; debilitating; horrible.

Comments:

[1055] Severe, cluster headaches are known to have caused suicide.

[1061] If anyone can give advice on how to calm myself when I get a cluster attack please let me know. I get suicidal and violent when I have one. Usually I am really laid back.

[1068] No one knows the pain of these headaches; it is hard for non-cluster sufferers to comprehend.

[1075] I can't imagine a worse pain than these headaches. The only word for them that I can think of is "devastating."

[1079] Unbearable!

[1081] My husband would rather die than have to endure the pain.

[1086] I don't mean to diminish the pain felt by migraine sufferers, but clusters are a whole 'nother ball game. I was told that I didn't know how to handle stress, or that I wasn't good at tolerating pain and had a very low pain threshold. I am personally convinced that cluster headache sufferers have very high pain thresholds.

[1087] Cluster headaches are so severe that they are only understood by other sufferers. They are devastating. The closest that I can come to describing them is having an ice pick stuck in my right eye and moved around about every five seconds. I won't give up; my father did 30 years ago. He took his life when they got too bad.

[1095-F] When I have an attack, I feel that no one understands how intense the pain is. Calling clusters headaches is a misnomer. The pain is worse than any I have experienced in my life, including childbirth and major surgery. My doctor told me that the pain level of clusters is right up there with terminal cancer pain.

[1100] Cluster headache is one of the most painful conditions known. I know this from experience after ten years of pain and numerous thoughts of suicide.

[1101] The pain is brutal. The only thing that's kept me going through my annual 30 day cycle was the knowledge that I could put up with a form of torture that would kill most men.

[1103] The pain is severe.

[1105] I have had a few cluster episodes where the pain was so intense that I passed out. I talked to a doctor and he told me that this could be the body's circuit breaker for pain. He said I shouldn't worry as long as other health indicators were okay.

[1106] The pain must be incredible because my father has a high pain tolerance and they literally bring him to his knees.

[1107] In my last bout of clusters, I twice had pain so severe that I went into shock. I awoke a short while later, lying on the floor. I was alone at home both times and found the experience quite frightening. The neurologist I consulted — the latest in a long line — assured me that this wasn't unheard of among cluster sufferers, and to his knowledge was not life-threatening.

[1116] Last month my husband and I were at the emergency room twice and the neurologist's office twice. While we were in the office the second time, my husband began having an attack and spent most of the time in the bathroom vomiting. I think the doctor was very surprised. I don't think they really understand the horrible pain cluster patients are experiencing.

[1119] If you can imagine a pair of pliers or vise grips getting a hold of one of your eyeballs and squeezing and twisting and tearing for about half an hour, then you have an idea of what a cluster headache typically feels like.

[1123] The agony is unbearable. My eye feels like a hot poker stabbing me. The first sign is my teeth starting to hurt. I know that the pain will not kill me, although I sometimes wish it would.

[1127-F] There is a very small warning period — perhaps a few seconds. Then the ache starts out slow and crescendos into a pain that is unexplainable unless you have experienced it. I have not reached a point of wanting to hurt myself to make it go away.

[1128] The pain is unbearable. No one knows that for three, four, five, or six hours the pain is so intense that you bang your head against the wall hoping to knock yourself out so that you won't experience it. No one knows that you wish someone would just shoot you to get it over with. They don't realize that no matter how you stand, sit, walk, move or hold your head that the pain just keeps on coming.

[1132] The pain is fierce. I did three tours in 'Nam, and was shot twice. The pain from the gun shot was a picnic compared to the clusters. My wife helps when she can, but even though I have a high pain threshold, these things make me act awful. I can't help it…it hurts!

[1134] I don't know anyone who wouldn't try anything in the midst of a cluster to stop it.

[1136] No one should have to go through the pain that these headaches give.

[1139] I suffer from deathly painful cluster migraines.

[1142-F] My friend suffers from cluster headaches. I have noticed when I am with her during really bad attacks that she passes out for about 15 to 40 seconds while in the middle of particularly intense pain. During this time she appears to have stopped breathing because when she comes to, she is gasping for air. During a bad attack of about 45 minutes she may pass out six or seven times. They are very frightening for me and I do not know if I should be racing her off to the hospital or not.

[1143] This "monster" must be subdued!

[1144] Let me preface this by saying that I am a migraine sufferer, as was my mother, and her father, so we are familiar with severe, intense headache pain. But I have never endured pain like I am about to describe. I am writing this for my 35 year old son who was diagnosed with cluster headaches eight years ago. This is pain we never thought possible! Needless to say, he could not stand the pain, which is usually in his right temple area, but recently sometimes involves both temple areas. He says the best way to describe the pain is as though bolts of lightening were constantly striking in the temples, radiating excruciating pain throughout the area over and over and over again.

[1145-F] No one can understand the terrible pain except other cluster sufferers. In medical texts, I've seen the pain of migraines called "severe" and the pain of clusters called "excruciating." I think that sums it up. Also, I've talked to women who have said that the pain of clusters was worse than the pain of childbirth.

[1146-F] To get rid of cluster pain I would cut off my right arm.

[1151] When I had my first cluster attack I actually thought my head was going to explode. I thought I had a brain tumor. I can't imagine the pain of being tortured as being worse than the pain experienced during cluster headache periods.

[1151] The pain is so intense, getting to sleep is impossible.

[1152] Horrible damn disease, these clusters. I treat lots of pain patients and this beats them all. Cluster headaches certainly have been effective in making me empathetic to those in pain.

[1154] Cluster headaches are not to be confused with migraine.

[1155] If you haven't had a cluster headache, you can't possibly understand what it feels like. These things are not headaches. Once, in the middle of a long drive, I had an attack. Try explaining to a cop why you are parked on the side of the road at nine o'clock in the morning with tears running down one side of your face and vomiting your guts up.

[1157] My neurologist said that his first cluster patient had been an avid gun collector. He sold his prized collection when the clusters started because he feared he would choose the ultimate path to relieve his pain forever.

[1158-F] It's difficult when you're banging your head against the wall hoping it will either kill you or at least knock you out.

[1160] I thought I had a brain tumor and was going to get a stroke. The pain is the only thing that is consistent. It is something few people could possibly fathom.

[1161] During a cluster attack I find that thrashing doesn't help. Neither does banging my head, screaming or yelling at my wife. I do have to sit up though, because laying down seems to aggravate it. No amount of pain, including childbirth, can match cluster pain. Over the years I have learned to calm myself and let the pain wash over me. The pain feels like a hot poker stuck in my right eyeball and another in my temple. Both pokers are trying to find each other and are turning my brain to hamburger. About eight years ago, I had a kidney stone stuck in my urethra; it hurt like hell. Laying on the bed, the doctor said it was one of the worst pains a man can experience other than something called cluster headaches, which he had only vaguely heard of. I assured him the clusters are far worse. Demerol killed the pain of the stone and let me sleep for three to four hours at a time, until they decided I wasn't going to pass the stone naturally so they went in with a tube to get it. Once, with the clusters getting so bad, I ended up in the emergency room. They gave me a shot of Demerol. My cluster subsided, but I wasn't sure if the shot really did anything or if the cluster was about to end on its own. I was real tired by then, having been fighting the pain off and on for eight hours. The hospital staff took me home. I crawled into bed and was asleep for only 45 minutes after getting the shot when another cluster brought me up off the sheets like a rocket. There is no comparison. If someone tells you that he knows what it feels like, ask him if anyone has ever reached into his eye socket and yanked out his eyeball. Unless he says yes, he doesn't know.

[1162] If you can describe the pain as tolerable then you are not having a cluster.

[1163-F] I describe the pain as "IT." This is my way of dealing with "IT." That way it's not a part of me but something that happens to me. Also, I can try to project the pain outward.

[1164] The pain of a cluster headache reaches the extremes of human suffering. Cluster is recurring purgatory.

[1166] Each headache would make me punch myself in the head, bang my head off walls, and pray to god to take my life. It felt like a knife was being plunged through my temple. It is the most severe pain imaginable.

[1167] The pain is so intense that a couple of times I thought that I was going to pass out. I have wished that I could fall unconscious just to get rid of the pain. The misery of the pain is hard if not impossible to imagine by people who do not suffer them. My co-workers, and even the boss, simply don't understand that a headache won't disappear with a couple of aspirin.

[1168] I find that I can't remember very many of my headaches. I think that I block out the memory.

[1170] My friend suffers from these dreadful headaches and cannot stand the pain.

[1171] Unless someone has experienced a cluster headache, it is impossible to know how you feel. I don't even know how I feel because each one seems to be more painful than I remembered. I think I forget how bad it hurts between headaches, as a type of defense. The pain is unlike anything else I have ever experienced. It is unlike a physical injury and is unmanageable. The agony is unbearable.

[1174] The pain is unbearable.

[1175] The pain is at the suicidal level.

[1179] God made minds; the devil made clusters.

[1181] Please help me; the pain is so bad.

[1182] Clusters cause an excruciating eye stab. The pain is intense, and afterwards the eye (usually the right) is extremely sore as if there were actual physical trauma.

[1184] Clusters cause very severe pain that is debilitating.

[1187-F] Unless someone has this condition, there is no understanding of the pain.

[1189-F] Unless you experience the pain, you can't possibly understand what it feels like. I think that I would kill myself if I had them chronically.

[1193] All of the severe pain that a migraine sufferer experiences in three to five days, a cluster sufferer experiences in one to two hours, up to ten times a day!

[1194] Intense pain.

[1197] I would wake up in the middle of the night coming out of a nightmare that I was in extreme pain. Well, it was no dream.

[1198] I am really afraid that my husband will not be able to withstand the pain much longer.

[1201] About five years ago during an attack, I realized that if I had a gun I would have used it on myself.

[1204] How can words possibly even begin to describe the pain?

[1211-F] These are headaches so bad that I can't work or exist!

[1212] I try not to panic. When I separate the fear from the pain, I find that the pain alone is easier to take.

[1213] Clusters cause intense pain.

[1216] Cluster sufferers know that they'll do anything to get by that "peak" period of pain. I was frightened today because the pain peaked for almost two hours. It's usually "only" about 45 minutes, so this is indeed scary.

[1217] My pain is tolerable right now. I am concerned that it will get worse as time goes on.

[1219-F] Sometimes my clusters are very intense, and sometimes I can deal with them.

[1222] I believe that the pain gets worse when the clusters take a year off. On these long periods the pain is more intense, and I had been ending up in the emergency room.

[1224] I go four or five days with just a mild pain. Gradually the pain will grow, and it will take too many pills to control it.

[1227-F] I awoke with the most severe headache I could imagine! I rolled back and forth in bed, covering my cries with my pillow.

[1229-F] I am thinking about breaking into a pharmacy and stealing Morphine, Demerol, and Dilaudid. I am also going to find a street connection for heroin. I'll just have to guess the strength of each dose to take.

[1233] Only another cluster headache sufferer can comprehend the level of pain we must deal with.

[1238-F The pain is so bad that I pray for death.

[1244] If you can tolerate it, it can't be a cluster.

[1245] Cluster pain has been described as much worse than the pain caused by bullet hits and traumatic amputations. It is a pain I could not wish even to my worst enemy.

[1246] A cluster headache is a very painful event. It causes horrible pain. I can't describe how bad the pain is if you haven't had one.

[1249] I have no memory, but my wife tells me that I lose consciousness during a bad attack. She assumes as I do that the intense pain causes this. People who get migraines tell me that they know exactly how I'm feeling. Bull! If they're experiencing the same pain, how can they lie still and motionless. I don't stop moving and screaming until the headache stops. There is no way to describe this. The pain feels like an alien creature trying to claw its way out of my head.

[1251] It is the most unbearable pain I've ever suffered.

[1254] I came within a hair of checking out when I was having three to six headaches a day. Clusters are the worst pain known.

[1255] It seems that there is a certain "quantity" of pain allocated to a cluster. If the cluster is shorter, the headaches are more severe. If it lasts longer, the headaches are not quite as severe. The pain is almost always a piercing stab in the right eye or between the right eye and the temple. It lasts with great intensity for several hours. One neurologist told me that the pain originates in the sphenopalatine ganglion.

[1257] I experience the pain as an animate being. After spending many ghoulish nights pacing a path into my living room rug, I've come to where I get these surrealistic fantasies of the pain being something tangible, with a life of its own. I talk to my pain as if it would make a difference. It doesn't, but helps pass those hellish moments. Without shared experience, there is no one who can understand this type of pain.

[1260] The pain is something I wouldn't wish on my worst enemy.

[1263-F] I am a college student and I just want the pain to stop because I can't deal with this much longer.

[1265-F] It is difficult to describe the pain to someone who has never experienced a cluster.

Effect on Life

A cluster headache is a disabling affliction that detrimentally affects many aspects of the victim's life. Unlike other headaches, one cannot simply "take a couple of aspirin" and continue with everyday events. In addition to the physical pain, this ailment impacts on emotions, marriage, finances, and worldly obligations. It clearly diminishes the quality of one's life.

Here is a list of typical comments made by exasperated cluster sufferers: I regularly miss work and other responsibilities; they're difficult on my spouse; I'm afraid to leave the house; I can't travel or go far from home; I live in constant fear of the next attack; It's embarrassing to have an attack in public; I'm afraid to go to sleep; I function for days on end with little or no rest; they're emotionally and financially draining; I am always depressed, anxious, and testy; I'm tired of fooling around with them; they're robbing my life.

Comments:

[1150] I am near the end of my rope.

[1052] Suffering from cluster headaches has been hell. Prior to finding relief, it was really bad going to work. I was lucky because I always got the headaches after work during the night, but I was always tired and depressed from the headaches the night before. This has been very difficult over the years on my wife, and I know how helpless she has felt. I know how helpless I have felt. In the early days, she drove me back and forth to the hospital to get shots, and kept the kids from bothering me during my headaches. I guess there wasn't much else she could do except to be understanding.

[1053] I am responsible for the completion of a given task over time, and whether I do this at home in my pajamas, or at the office, is of little concern to my employer. It has been terribly important to find jobs like this so that my attacks escape notice. This has given me the opportunity to deal with them on my own terms, in my own time. I do not tell my employers that I have a medical problem because I do not expect them to understand. I don't understand what is happening to me, so why should they? Once in a while, but rarely, these people witness a strong attack. I try to let them know that 1) This has happened before and that I know what is happening to me, 2) It has nothing to do with them, and 3) What I most need to do after an attack is to repair to a quiet private place, by myself, and resume work (or whatever) on the next day. I try not to be afraid of the attacks. Resisting the attacks makes them markedly worse. I try to trust that I have sufficient internal resources to face what is happening and to maintain my composure.

[1054] It is very difficult for people to live their lives with this condition. My husband gets a cluster once or twice a year for a month to two months, and during these clusters he regularly misses work and other obligations. Of course, bosses, co-workers, and friends don't understand. I wonder how other cluster sufferers' significant others cope with this. I just try to be as understanding as possible, and there for him, but I always feel inadequate.

[1061] These things are so debilitating. I can't work or attend my college classes because they come at any time.

[1068-F] It is embarrassing for my wife to have a cluster attack in public or around family members.

[1070] I have learned to cope as well as I believe is possible.

[1071] My clusters have had a devastating effect on my life. Without them, I am much more productive, and a lot more happy.

[1072] I am going through a really weird experience caused by a high dose of drugs to control my clusters. My wife is scared.

[1075] I'd be sitting in class when one side of my head would get severe jabs from my eye all the way to my shoulder. I would flinch and try to push on my forehead really hard to make it go away.

[1095] I live in constant fear of the next cluster attack — not knowing when it will hit or whether I'll be driving at the time.

[1101] When I had clusters in high school people thought I was on drugs, and many a day had been ruined.

[1102] I am afraid to sleep knowing that I will wake up from the pain of another headache. I would give important parts of my anatomy for a good night of sleep.

[1112] My husband had to quit his job, and is functioning during the day only because he is a strong man. I am not so strong. This terrible problem is about to do us in.

[1114] I told my colleague that a cluster cycle was on its way and that I could get easily irritated during the next couple of weeks.

[1117] The clusters are so bad that I get sick, sweat, and get an upset stomach. I requested Social Security Insurance because I lost my job from being sick with these headaches all the time.

[1128] I tried to go to work today, but as soon as I got there I knew it was futile. I was walking around like a zombie and just couldn't function. Migraine sufferers can lay down most of the time. I wish I could for five minutes. In a few hours I get to look forward to another night of hell with no sleep, and if I can possibly go into work tomorrow, some idiot may offer me a sleeping pill. They just don't understand.

[1140] Clusters seriously interfere with my life, and I'm tired of fooling around with them.

[1145-F] I'm unable to work during cluster episodes, so I'm out on disability. When a cycle starts, I go to my supervisor and explain what's happening. I used to feel embarrassed and ashamed when I got these attacks. I felt like something was wrong with me, and I didn't tell anyone in the workplace. Years ago, I decided to come out of the closet. This has helped enormously. Sometimes, people at work say, "That's so weird!" And I say, "Yeah, isn't it strange." Now my co-workers are supportive and curious. Hell, I'd be curious, too. It is weird. Also, I've decided to give myself a gift at work. Since my attacks last for one month, I go on short-term disability for the month. (I can do this without putting my job in jeopardy.) One of the most nerve-wracking aspects of this is wondering if the episode will truly end when they're "supposed to." I mean, how does my head know when to quit this nonsense so I can get back to my real life?

[1155] I want and need sleep, but I know what will happen about 30 minutes after I go to sleep. I don't even sleep with my wife when I'm in a cluster period because she needs her sleep.

[1156-F] When I'm in cycle I fear going to sleep at night. I am already worried about this coming up again, but I plan on having my arsenal of treatments ready. I want to have another baby, but I was not allowed to get pregnant this year because of all the strong medication I was taking. My doctors want me to get pregnant and give birth between cluster seasons.

[1161] If I can get a few hours of sleep in between the pain, I may be able to function the next day. Last evening, at a very important company affair, I had an attack and had to leave. I explained the situation to my boss; my company is very understanding. I have to decide whether to cancel a planned trip next week and chalk up the nonrefundable air fare to the pain devil. It's a good thing I don't operate heavy machinery, but my job does require a good deal of thought and decisions. Christmas won't be too jolly for me this year. I can't wait for it to be over because that will be a month away, and hopefully my headaches will be gone.

[1162] The anxiety I feel immediately before and during the cluster season is almost as bad as the actual pain of the headache.

[1168] When I have a cluster headache, I can barely bring myself to think, much less speak.

[1172] The past two weeks have been hell. The disruption of my life is depressing. The anxiety from having them may cause another round, and I will not function normally for at least a month.

[1174] Sleep deprivation is the untold story. When you rarely sleep for several weeks, it really affects your quality of life.

[1181] I live in fear.

[1182] The cost and disappointment when there's no relief or improvement becomes exasperating.

[1193] I'm scared to even leave the house because I don't know when one will hit. They aren't something that you want to have in public. People just don't understand.

[1204] I have endured the skepticism of co-workers and bosses who can't begin to imagine the debilitating effects of a "simple" headache — not to mention the agony of family members who witness the effects and are helpless to intervene.

[1207] I go into a state of panic before the "season" starts. Will they come? When? Once I'm in a cluster season, I have a hard time leading a normal life because I can't travel, go too far from home, or do my normal hobbies in case of attacks. During an attack I'm unable to work for at least one hour, and I just lean over my desk trying to get through it. My job is very accommodating.

[1208] I feel testy, weak, and unable to relax.

[1223] I don't know how much longer I can take it, so I am also on drugs for anxiety and depression.

[1247] I'm just about ready to give up. I'm drained emotionally and financially.

Triggers

Although no one knows what causes a cluster headache, some things are thought to provoke the condition. These may be referred to as cluster "triggers." There is some consensus regarding a few of these triggers but little agreement about most of the others.

Cluster triggers are unusual in that they do not seem to induce the affliction when the subject is not in the midst of a cycle. In other words, a certain food may be acceptable to ingest for several months, only to cause a headache once a cluster episode has begun.

Alcohol, smoking, and relaxation (including sleep, as well as the let-down that follows stress and heavy exercise), appear to be the most conspicuous of the cluster triggers. Here is a list of other potential triggers, presented in an approximate order matching the number of times they were considered to cause an attack: seasonal factors (including variable changes in daylight); weather variations (including changes in altitude and barometric pressure); chemical and hormonal imbalances (including serotonin levels, circadian rhythms, disruptive sleep patterns, sleep apnea, and low blood oxygen); allergies; toxic food (including nitrites, MSG, and food containing trace amounts of detrimental substances); specific foods; food in general (eating anything); certain over-the-counter drugs; perfumes and other odors; trauma to the body. A summary of these possible triggers may be found in the appendix on page 75.

Comments:

[1050] I am a recovering alcoholic, and suffered from cluster headaches for many years. One thing I found out real quick was that alcohol and clusters do not mix. Alcohol made the headaches last longer, and they were more severe. Whenever I was having cluster attacks I abstained from alcohol completely.

[1052] I stopped smoking 13 years ago but the clusters continued.

[1055] I knew that nitrites and MSG can trigger migraines, but I just recently considered that they could effect cluster headaches. I guess it makes sense, though, if the monosodium glutamate and nitrites expand blood vessels. Alcohol expands blood vessels, and alcohol certainly is an immediate trigger for clusters. I think nitrites (and nitrates?) may be found in some cheeses, hot dogs, and wine. I will certainly monitor this during future cluster periods.

[1057] I have noted on two occasions that my expected episode was either broken or delayed when I was under emotional duress.

[1058] I am a jogger. During a cluster spell I will get a headache within ten minutes at the end of my run.

[1061] This first time I ever had clusters was when I came home from the Army. I had just started smoking at the time. I feel that allergies may be responsible, but all my doctors say no.

[1063] After years of suffering, I had a sleep study run and it was found that I suffered from sleep apnea. The sleep study indicated a slight decline of oxygen in my bloodstream while I slept. It was this decrease that was thought to cause my waking with a headache.

[1066] According to my doctor, attacks often occur when the body relaxes. This would explain the fact that during a cluster period I can never get through an evening without attacks.

[1077] My headaches seem to be histamine activated. I may be having an allergic reaction to something in the air. I have had many different allergy tests, but the clusters still remain a mystery.

[1078] Cluster headaches have been caused by nitrites. I was able to trace most of my worst attacks to times when I was in cities with high levels in their water.

[1080] Drinking alcohol and smoking is not a good idea during the cluster period.

[1081] There doesn't seem to be a reason for my husband's cycle with clusters. We have been married for 17 years, and have maintained the same jobs. Nothing has changed in our lifestyles. The clusters are not brought on by stress, but there does seem to be a link with alcohol and certain foods, but only when he is in a cycle.

[1086] Narcotics can trigger an acute cluster due to their "relaxing" effect, which almost killed me when a doctor injected Demerol for my clusters. It prolonged the acute attack, dragging it out over six hours, when mine are usually diminished in 30 to 90 minutes.

[1087] I don't get clusters during hard exercise. They never seem to appear, even when I'm normally getting them four or five times a day, until after I've cooled down from the strenuous workout. I've gotten them during light activity more than once.

[1088] My clusters coincide with stressful periods of my life.

[1091] Eating anything, especially red meat, would start the two hour cycle. Beer and red wine — forget it.

[1092] I am convinced that alcohol will almost certainly trigger a headache. Beer is the worst, followed by wine.

[1095-F] Insomnia usually precipitates another attack.

[1101] What blew me away was when the doctors said my clusters were related to the change in light. For 18 years my headaches came near Easter. They said it had nothing to do with the holiday, but with the change in the hours of light complicated by the leap to daylight savings time. I confirmed their theory. Only once had a cycle hit other than in May. That was the year I traveled from Asia to Australia in January. I do a lot of international travel, but that move was the only winter to summer transition, and it brought on bad cluster headaches.

[1104] Ever since I quit smoking over two years ago, and virtually stopped drinking alcohol (I still like a drink before dinner now and then), I have only had one cycle, which was incredibly mild. I really feel that quitting smoking was the key.

[1109] Alcohol is the first thing to be eliminated when a cycle begins. Spicy and fried foods also seem to bring them on. I usually go with a completely bland diet at the onset of a cycle. I think caffeine has actually helped me through an attack.

[1121] I went to an allergy specialist who determined that I had several severe "environmental" allergies such as ragweed, pollen, and dust, even though I did not show any traditional signs such as watery eyes and a runny nose. We concluded that a year of allergy shots might be worth a try to see if my allergic reactions were appearing as severe headaches that had been misdiagnosed as clusters. After the year of allergy shots, I made it through the first fall season in 15 years without experiencing a "cluster" headache. I stopped the allergy shots for a year, and this year I am suffering from my headaches once again. Although I am convinced that allergies are, at least in part, the cause of my headaches, my doctor claims that there is no documented evidence to suggest that allergies cause headaches like mine.

[1122-F] After I moved from Arizona to California — to an area with a high incidence of allergic reactions — I began having "sinus" headaches. After another year, they began increasing in frequency and severity to the degree that I sought medical advice and was told they were cluster migraines. I don't correlate them with allergies, though; I think they may be caused by weather changes, from high to low pressure, or from low to high pressure. I have since moved again to a climate which is damper and where weather changes are more frequent. After several years without anything other than an occasional headache, I am again noticing an increase in occurrence and severity, mainly during the "rainy" season. I don't believe I am imagining the connection, although there may be other factors that I'm not aware of.

[1126] Things that trigger my clusters: smells like old coffee, perfume, tobacco smoke, and smoke from a wood fire. I have not found any foods that trigger a headache, but booze always does.

[1133] Being a coffeeholic (4 to 6 cups of coffee or 12 cans of Cola) is probably what caused my clusters. I've noticed that when I drink coffee early in the day, I pay for it later with increased pain and more headache occurrences.

[1136] I've been in high altitudes, low altitudes, hot weather and cold weather. It doesn't make a difference.

[1143] I've had clusters while living in three different states, so I don't think they're related to the daylight I am exposed to.

[1145-F] Clusters are related to changes in light. Do not drink or smoke, and keep your sleep cycle the same every night. If I change my sleep pattern I'll get a headache.

[1154] My sleep patterns, food and caffeine intake do not change during a cluster season to warrant this type of reaction. Cluster headaches are not caused by caffeine or caffeine withdrawal. I've had both types of headache, and there's no comparison.

[1155] I don't eat after six in the evening.

[1156-F] My cycles come when the Arizona monsoons arrive. They are highly charged electrical storms, with little rain, fierce winds, and a big change in barometric pressure. I lived in California twice and did not suffer at all. But as soon as I returned to Phoenix and the monsoons arrived, my headaches returned. One year, there were no storms in Phoenix, and I didn't get the headaches.

[1157] There is a definite connection between alcohol and clusters — in the most minute amounts. Artificial flavorings, like vanilla extract, contain alcohol. I'm convinced a cluster was induced by eating a glazed donut. Citrus, I believe, is another culprit. Read the ingredients on prepared foods; lemon juice is used a lot.

[1160] I wonder if clusters are related to changes in daylight. I work inside all day long and rarely get to see the sun. I also read a story once about a fighter pilot who got clusters when he flew on long trips. That probably relates to the change in air pressure.

[1164] I don't agree with the notion that dilated blood vessels in the head cause cluster headache. Nobody can explain why constriction or dilation of blood vessels should cause pain. After all, blood vessels routinely constrict and dilate without pain. I believe the pain is generated by a disturbance in normal neurochemistry, and is not due to any physical changes or damage. Changes in blood vessels are the result, not the cause, of the neurochemical disturbance. For the same reason, I do not believe odors precipitate or "trigger" headaches; rather, I think it is the headache that causes odors to seem more powerful than usual. Sensory disturbances, when they occur, generally precede onset of the headache.

[1166] My cluster headaches are not related to caffeine or caffeine withdrawal.

[1167] I usually drink four to five cans of Coke per day. Last spring I decided to reduce my volume of Coke. Soon thereafter, I had a severe cycle of cluster pains which seemed to last an eternity. Coke contains caffeine. I wonder if caffeine withdrawal triggered my cluster, or whether it would have come anyway that spring. Also, my clusters appeared following a period of severe stress at the office. Once I could relax, my cycle started. I also suspected that something in my diet had to be the cause. Although I avoided cheese, alcohol, and chocolates, like the neurologist suggested, it simply did not work.

[1169] I have known three other males who have clusters. Including myself, they all smoke. I also think clusters are seasonal related. They seem to be affected by barometric changes.

[1171] Alcohol is a trigger. I even switched to a water-based after-shave. Airplane trips should be avoided during a cluster cycle.

[1172] I get cluster headaches whenever the barometric pressure changes drastically, especially when a high pressure system is passing through, or when it clears after a storm. Usually 30.00 and rising indicates definite problems to come.

[1173] I read about a study that linked clusters with the change in seasons. It found that the highest incidence of cluster episodes occurs around the time of the summer and winter solstices. There seems to be a link to circadian rhythms and the hypothalamus.

[1174] Blood sugar and serotonin levels may affect clusters. Here is a list of foods that may trigger an episode: 1) MSG; 2) alcohol of any kind, especially red wine or beer; 3) sodium nitrates, found in many cold cuts, sausage, and cured meats; 4) nuts, especially peanut butter; 5) table salt; 6) large quantities of whole milk. Here are some other cluster triggers: seasonality, or being near in time to the change of seasons. Smoking is said to have an adverse effect. Odors, including gasoline, some perfumes, hair sprays and other aerosols. Several doctors recommend: 1) don't drink or smoke; 2) if it's cheap and tasty, don't eat it. Paradoxically, both nicotine, which constricts the arteries, and alcohol, which dilates them, trigger cluster headaches. The exact connection between these substances and cluster attacks is not known. I also noticed that the frequency of attacks decreased when I had some of my mercury fillings removed.

[1180] I suffer the most during periods when my schedule prevents me from exercising on a regular basis.

[1183] I am sensitive to seafood and some cheeses.

[1188] Almost all headaches are reactions of the brain and nervous system to substances that have been inhaled or ingested. Most headaches are caused by casein, the main protein in milk and dairy foods, chocolate, MSG (monosodium glutamate), or Aspartame, found in many diet foods.

[1197] Clusters seem to occur during the fall and spring — when the amount of sunlight is changing the fastest. This may indicate a problem with serotonin levels in the brain. Another cluster trigger is staying up too late or disrupting sleep patterns. This may be related to serotonin imbalances as well. I also think that bright video screens, like sitting in front of your computer for prolonged periods, may contribute to the disruption of sleep patterns.

[1203] Because cluster headaches occur predominantly within males, a chemical or hormonal imbalance may be at the root of the problem. The foods we ingest are very important and have been proved to influence mood, athletic performance, and chemical processes. Pesticides and non-organic meat and dairy products contain chemicals and hormones that affect the body in unique ways. Cows are fed growth hormones, and are given antibiotics for ailments that regularly plague the poor heifers. When you eat a cheese pizza, or enjoy your frozen yogurt made with non-organic milk, you are ingesting the chemicals and hormones that were given to the cow. These may upset the delicate balance necessary to regulate the body. It is possible that these "poisons" accumulate in one's system until there is an overload. Then the adrenal glands (responsible for regulating chemical and hormonal processes) go haywire. Blood oxygen levels may rise and fall, the "poisoned" hypothalamus may alter sleep patterns, and the optic capillaries and nerves — the body's weak links — may be detrimentally affected. Extreme pain is the result.

[1205-F] The clusters that I used to get everyday were brought on by the fluorescent lights at work.

[1212] I believe that seasonal factors are involved. Serotonin is linked to daily and seasonal cycles. Unusually high exposure to sunlight during an episode can make the nighttime attacks more intense. My latest attacks began the day I moved into an office with fluorescent lights. Many cluster sufferers are smokers. Quitting tobacco may make the attacks less frequent but more intense when they do occur due to the loss of the vasoconstricting effects of nicotine. Low blood oxygen levels seem to be implicated in cluster attacks. High testosterone could also be correlated with clusters, especially considering the almost exclusively male incidence.

[1213] Cluster sufferers should keep a diary to detect triggers.

[1214] My colleague's cluster headaches began when he moved from southern Europe to Sweden, where seasonal differences in daylight hours are much more evident.

[1217] I do not drink coffee or take anything which may contain caffeine except when the cluster has already appeared. Stress makes me feel a cluster aura — a vague sensation that a cluster pain is imminent. Sometimes, when stress is intolerable, I end up with a cluster cycle. The cluster appears when the stress is going away.

[1218-F] Some of my worst headaches occur during alcohol intake.

[1231] My new cycle started ten days after my wife left me. After she left, my diet slipped to include junk food filled with nitrites and preservatives. The first week I was too depressed to go out of the house. The next couple of weeks were spent working odd hours. So, stress, food, sunlight, and sleep cycles could all be implicated. I'm now trying to reverse all of the above and see what happens.

[1232] I was diagnosed with stress tics at around the same time as my cluster headaches started to appear. Sometimes my clusters come when I am in a stressful period, but I don't believe they are stress related because they also come when I am completely relaxed and in non-stressful situations. They even wake me at night.

[1236] If I go without breakfast and lunch, and my blood sugar drops, I'll get an aura then a headache.

[1239] Trauma to the body may be one factor related to the onset of cluster headaches. I've suffered through these since I had sinus surgery. I believe there are triggers unique to each individual. My first occurrences were in college when I was under a lot of stress.

[1240] In North Carolina, where I live, I was clustering like crazy. They stopped when I traveled to Boston for a week, and resumed as soon as I returned. So climate or allergies may be a component.

[1248] I try to avoid foods with nitrites as preservatives. I also avoid water that is high in nitrates. This is a common problem with water supplies in the Midwest. This has not done away with my clusters, but has made them much easier to tolerate.

[1252-F] My headaches usually occur in the afternoon when I start to relax. This is also beer time for me. I noticed that on Saturday I had a beer earlier in the day than usual, and the daily headaches started earlier. Sunday, no beer — no headache! I'm skeptical about medications that treat the cause of headaches as vascular. The vascular changes could easily be caused by something else.

[1255] In the early years my clusters could be triggered by strong odors, like perfume or cologne, especially if I was in a closed space, like a theater or auditorium.

[1262] Alcohol in any form is an immediate trigger. A sip of wine will set me off in less than ten minutes. This also means avoiding most shaving creams, mouthwash, and cologne. Non-prescription drugs may also trigger an attack. I took over-the-counter pills to improve my memory and suffered from the worst and longest peak period I have ever had. There seem to be so many other triggers that I have given up trying to avoid them.

[1266] I live near the coast, and years ago I made a correlation with eating shrimp and cluster bouts that followed within hours or days of consumption. I think that the offending batches of shrimp had been harvested after ingesting a particular toxin, which triggered the physical sequence of events that led to my cluster episodes. All of my bouts occurred when outbreaks of toxic "red tide" algae blooms took place. I stopped eating shrimp and went seven years without a cluster. Also, my wife claims that I often stop breathing for five or ten seconds, even while awake. I wonder if this can cause low blood oxygen levels which initiate some of the attacks, especially the ones while asleep.

Treatment and Relief

In this chapter, cluster headache sufferers offer candid input regarding their strategies for coping with this enigmatic ailment. More than 70 different treatments were tried, with varying results. These included over-the-counter medications, prescription drugs, natural remedies, dietary modifications, and an assortment of other unique attempts at achieving cluster relief.

A complete analysis of treatment results is presented in the appendix starting on page 75. However, some general observations will be noted at this point: 1) No one seems to know what causes a cluster headache. Therefore, prevention in not yet a viable option. 2) Many sufferers reported that a treatment that was effective for one or more cluster attacks or cluster episodes, often proved to be ineffective on future headaches. Dosages had to be increased as the headaches became more severe or as the body gained a tolerance to the medication. 3) Treatments that were effective for some sufferers proved to be worthless to others. 4) Several sufferers voiced their concerns about the potentially dangerous side effects of Imitrex, Prednisone, Lithium, Sansert, and other medications.

Comments:

[1050] I consumed thousands of pain killers with absolutely no relief. My doctor then prescribed Cafergot, and it worked, but only if taken before the headache started. The problem with Cafergot is that you are only supposed to take six or seven a week. This is unrealistic for clusters which can occur multiple times a day. Needless to say, I ended up taking many more than what was recommended, which was kind of scary to me, but I had to have relief from that devastating, disabling pain.

[1051] The only relief I get is from taking a hot shower and letting the water spray on the back of my neck and top of my head. I'm not sure if this has any benefit other than distracting me while the session time goes by. I discovered the other night that putting my head between my knees cut the time of the attacks to about five minutes. My eye still tears and my left nostril still runs, but five minutes instead of 20 to 30 is a relief. A new doctor I'm seeing put me on Prednisone, a steroid drug. (Yes, the one on the evening news that was dissolving some guy's hips.) He assured me that was an isolated case, and that side effects like that come from long exposure. My dosage is 60mg per day for five days, 40mg for days

6 through 10, 20mg for days 11 through 15, then stop. After my fourth day of 60mg I did experience some relief. Going through a day with only a slight tight feeling in my head is a far cry from my left side wanting to give birth to an alien creature trying to claw it's way out! But Prednisone is not a "cycle stopper." It just alters the nature of the headaches. The time and intensity have changed.

[1052] A few years ago I accidentally found a combination of drugs that completely subdues all headaches during the cluster period. I take 20mg of Prozac and 2mg of Sansert twice a day (12 hours apart). Neither medication by itself is effective, but the combination works miracles for me. I also have oxygen standing by, but I only need it when I have to go off the medication to see if the cluster has ended yet or not. This combination has been effective through three different episodes over the past five years.

[1054] My husband has not had a headache in two days since he started taking Tavist 1. He knows that he was not at the end of his cluster when he began taking it. He normally takes Lithium when he senses the cluster coming on, although he's not really sure if it ever did anything. He uses Imitrex for the pain, although he gets severe rebound headaches from it. His first try with Imitrex was two years ago, using the shot. It was a miracle, the very first thing that stopped the pain. Now that it is in tablet form, he's trying it again. It seemed to work at first, but now it isn't working as well, so he obtained a larger dosage, and is getting rebound headaches again. They are worse than the initial headache. Imitrex is good for situations where he must immediately get rid of the pain, like when he's at work. He's also tried Ergotamine, Sansert, and Prednisone, among other things, none of which have ever really helped.

[1055] I use Imitrex for my cluster headaches. It stops them within five minutes. However, after using the Imitrex tablets for several days, I developed rebound headaches and began having the attacks at night. I used Prednisone during my last cluster cycle and it worked miraculously. I was left with slight burning sensations in my temple, instead of the normal excruciating and incapacitating cluster attack. The doctors and books are not very clear on what exactly happens with long term corticosteroid usage. I used it for two weeks, which the doctor said should not cause any problems. The only side effect I have found regular mention of is immune system suppression. That sounds bad enough to me.

[1057] I found that Demerol works quickly and effectively during the early and waning periods. To deal with the peak period I've tried Fiorinal with Codeine, Ergodryl, and Prednisone. Nothing stopped the peak period attacks. I hardly slept during the week I took Prednisone. (I have an acquaintance whose brittle, crumbling hip bones have been attributed to two years of Prednisone use.) Find a knowledgeable, sympathetic doctor, preferably a neurologist, and then, through trial and error, find the medication that will help you deal with the pain.

[1059] Given subcutaneously, Sumatriptan as an autoinjection (automatic injection by pressing a button on a special pen) will relieve most attacks within 10 to 15 minutes.

[1060] Oxygen is the most effective and least expensive method to stop cluster headaches.

[1063] I have been using a continuous positive airway pressure machine while I sleep. I have fewer and less severe headaches as a result. For the few that still occur, I have been using 25mg Imitrex tablets with success. They are not as quick as the injectable form, but I do find relief within one-and-a-half hours. The tablets sell for around $10 a pop, while the injectable form runs around $35.

[1064] I've tried lots of different drugs: Prednisone, Ergotamine, Verapamil, Imitrex, and anti-depressants. Most work initially, but start to lose their effectiveness. It's almost as if the only way to get out of a cluster is to at some point experience the pain. Imitrex works sometimes, although not nearly as well as when I first started using it. In fact, if I don't get the Imitrex down at the very first sign of a headache, it does nothing at all. Over the years, Verapamil has been the most effective at treating the headaches. If I didn't take it, I would get the headaches every day. When I do take it, I only get the headaches when I'm in a really serious part of the cycle. My doctor also gave me Stadol, a pain killer that comes as a nasal spray. It doesn't get rid of the headache, but it takes enough of the edge off so that I'm not banging my head against the wall. It's fast, and expensive...just like Imitrex. Thank god for insurance.

[1068-F] My wife started her season two months ago and held the attacks at bay with minimal medication: 10mg Prozac and 5mg Prednisone. Five days ago they returned in earnest. She gets a headache two hours after falling asleep, so we have Imitrex 50mg tablets, and she takes them before she goes to sleep. Now she gets four hours of sleep before a cluster comes on.

[1070] As soon as I begin sensing the aura of a cluster cycle coming on, I take Wygraine and Verapamil, one each before every meal. As long as I keep the dosage up, I don't have headaches. I also keep an oxygen bottle nearby during the cycle, just in case.

[1071] About a year ago, a psychiatrist prescribed Elavil, which works both as an anti-depressant and, in my case, an effective remedy for the clusters. I take 100mg at bedtime, and it has the added benefit of helping me to sleep.

[1072] Injectable Sumatriptan always works for me. The pills never work. Before this, I tried Deltasone, Inderal, Ergotamine, and others, with no prophylactic efficiency.

[1073] When I was first diagnosed, the emergency room doctor suspected clusters and gave me oxygen; the relief came in about five minutes. Imitrex injections have worked consistently as well.

[1074] I've tried many different prescriptions, some good, some very bad. The best relief was oxygen inhaled for ten minutes. It worked miracles during the first cluster period, but stopped being effective as time passed. Since then, the best prevention has been from Verapamil and Prednisone. For relief during an attack, an intramuscular injection of DHE 45 is very effective, and usually diminishes the pain to a bearable level. Something new that I've tried this session is Stadol. It's a nasal spray for pain relief, and works very quickly. The combination of the DHE 45 and Stadol during an attack has been a godsend to me.

[1076] Oxygen is the best treatment for short term relief. Sansert and Verapamil will also work for short periods of time. Lithium may be used, but have your blood tested regularly.

[1077] I have tried many different things. For relief I take Sansert and oxygen. This has worked for me for the past five years.

[1078] I have been buying water treated by reverse osmosis, and have noticed a significant decrease in the frequency and severity of my attacks.

[1080] I have been studying this for 15 years. The best medicine is an Imitrex injection. Oxygen is good but not always successful. I wish there were a natural remedy but I haven't found one.

[1081] My husband has tried everything. Sometimes, if he pays attention to the signals that his body sends him, he can stop the cluster by drinking coffee. He also uses stress relief techniques to concentrate on breathing and transmitting heat to his extremities. Currently, the winner is Imitrex shots. My husband wants to say that Imitrex works, although he doesn't like giving himself the shots and worries about the long term effects. I can't stand the drug because of its long term maintenance with lots of side effects.

[1082] I take 10 liters per minute for half an hour or less, and this stops the headache. With the oxygen I can return to my old self in a short while. My insurance covers everything: the tanks, valves, and the mask. An oxygen company delivers the tanks right to my door. I keep a large "M" tank at home, and I have a small portable "E" tank that I travel with. It's not a cure, but it sure makes me feel that I have some control over this horrible pain.

[1083] A natural remedy of 2000mg of calcium plus 1000mg of magnesium has helped to relieve the intensity of my headaches. The chelated form is best. This combination is supposed to control muscle contractions and transmit nerve impulses to the brain. Although it upsets my stomach a little, the trade-off is worth it.

[1086] I started taking Ergotamine, with very good results. I've had two days where I was able to prevent attacks before they started. I tried deep breathing exercises and have had limited success. The hyperventilation effect gives me a different kind of headache, on top of the cluster, but the cluster did subside somewhat. I believe strongly in chiropractic treatments for many ailments, but not for clusters. Demerol put me out of control so that I could not use any of the biofeedback coping methods that I had developed. Cafergot (caffeine plus Ergotamine) helps, and for several years I relied upon Sansert along with over-the-counter caffeine (No-Doz, etc.) plus sickening strong coffee (four heaping tablespoons with warm tap water) to make an attack go away. This coffee technique is handy if you're stuck somewhere with no other relief in sight. It takes 10 to 15 minutes to work, and it is disgusting to drink, but you'd be surprised at what you'll do to make an acute attack go away. I also use Ergotamine suppositories at bedtime to prevent attacks that sneak up on you about two hours after falling asleep.

[1087] I can't count the nights I woke up with an "ice pick" stuck in my right eye and spent the next hour in the shower with hot water hitting my face. I'm in the middle of another episode, but seem to be controlling them this time using Fiorinal. When I can get a couple into my system right at the onset, it seems to work. They do cause fatigue and slow thinking though. Other drugs don't seem to help, but who knows how much worse the clusters would be without them.

[1088] Valium worked very well for 16 years, then it stopped working. Elavil worked but made me so groggy that I couldn't function the next day. My doctor switched me to Cafergot, which has worked nicely with no side effects, although I am concerned about the long-term effects. It seems to work best as a preventative, taken two or three hours before the onset of a headache. When I take it after the headache has gained a foothold, I'll suffer up to six hours. If I don't take it at all, the headache doesn't go away. But in the last few days the clusters have started anew with a vengeance.

[1089] I'll use oxygen at eight liters per minute with Percodan, because oxygen won't work by itself. Prednisone stopped the headaches until I got to one pill a day, then the headaches returned.

[1090] My neurologist prescribed Prednisone 80mg for five days. Clearly, the headaches are less painful and the episodes are shorter. I used calcium channel blockers during my last three episodes. I take Calan 240mg slow release until the headache episode is gone.

[1091] I have been through the gamut of medications from Sansert and Cafergot to beta-blockers, with no permanent results other than severe abdominal distress. I even tried not eating all day until after work. It got me through the day but not the evening. Recently my doctor prescribed oxygen. Amazing! My headache was gone in 15 to 20 minutes. It came back every two hours. Last week I tried Tavist 1 — one every 12 hours. So far, no more headaches. I'm keeping the oxygen close by just in case.

[1092] I've tried Sansert, which prevented headaches during the first two clusters, but seemed to diminish in efficacy after that. Sansert was one scary medicine. My veins ached around my arms and legs. My specialist had also warned me of its potentially deadly side effects — liver disease, scarring of the stomach lining, etc. So I did not want to stay on Sansert, especially when its effectiveness was waning. Then a neurologist put me on Isoptin (Verapamil), a calcium channel blocker, which worked great for the first cluster, but not as well the next couple of times. When I reduced the dosage too fast, I had rebound headaches that were worse than my normal headaches. Oxygen is excellent if you can use it as soon as you feel the onset of a cluster. My specialist told me to use it sitting up rather than lying down. I do seven liters per minute, for about ten minutes, and the headache goes away completely.

[1093] Here is what I have been prescribed over the years: Valium, Elavil, Demerol (oral and injection), Seconal, Fiorinal, Cafergot, Midrin, Darvon, and biofeedback therapy. Few were able to help me, although a couple did provide temporary relief. I quit taking regular medication; here is how I deal with them now: At the very first sign, I get in the shower and set the "shower massage" to heavy pulse, and progressively set the water temperature to as hot as I can bear. Then I move the pulse stream over my eye in a back and forth motion. Sitting on the shower floor takes the pressure off my body and prevents dizziness. It is not unusual for me to take three or four showers like this a night. The headache normally goes away within 10 to 20 minutes, or at least decreases in intensity to a level that is tolerable. The key is to catch it early. I recognize that this is only a short term solution, but it gets me through the night with a few hours of sleep.

[1094-F] I've tried it all. Some things worked for awhile but the headaches always found a way around them. Be cautious with Sansert. Long term use can lead to severe kidney problems. I did not find it effective, and the doctor finally gave up and sent me to an acupuncturist. Prednisone always reduced the frequency of the headaches but I invariably had breakthrough headaches at each step-down, and ended up on it for two months. I gained weight and experienced depression after the cycle. I tried Imitrex with great success. A shot of Imitrex will take the headache, eye tearing, nasal congestion, light sensitivity, and nausea away within twelve minutes. It has worked for me for three years now. Oxygen has provided dramatic and almost immediate relief for other sufferers.

[1095-F] I've tried every regimen doctors have prescribed, only to suffer side effects from the drugs, while still getting my headaches. I have tried Prednisone, Elavil, Sansert, beta blockers, and channel blockers, with some relief but no cure. Lidocaine liquid on a long Q tip, inserted into the nostril on the affected side, helps to numb the sphenopalatine ganglion (the source of the cluster) but doesn't touch the temple or eye pain. The only thing that really works is an Imitrex injection — I'll be pain-free in six minutes — but it's quite expensive, not to mention the dangerous side effects. I am now on Paxil. Even though I still get the headaches once a week, the pain intensity and length of time are reduced by about 40 percent, but they are still unbearable because I bang my head and can't stay still when they hit. I also take Hydrocodone, which sometimes takes the edge off the pain, enabling me to relax and do deep breathing. It's hard to do, but if you can take your conscious focus off the headache, and concentrate on breathing in, holding for six seconds, then breathing out, it does seem to alleviate the pain somewhat.

[1097] Verapamil is the only drug I have taken which prevents the headaches. I took this, and after a few days they stopped. However, my next cluster came earlier than usual, and I am now taking a double dose of Verapamil and Nortriptyline. This prevents pain.

[1098] I have tried Verapamil and didn't get any relief. I've tried 15 or 20 other miracle drugs, and none of them were effective.

[1099] I tried most of the standard treatments. Other than Lithium, which has bad side effects, Calan is the only other treatment that has worked. I'm not an advocate of Imitrex injections because although the headaches were stopped within five minutes, each subsequent headache was more intense than the last one. I had a total of eight injections (at $120 a shot) and found that the seventh produced the worst cluster I have ever had!

[1100] Imitrex probably saved my life. I had to really work on my HMO doctor to get it, it is very expensive, and you will continue to have attacks, but with the injections and home oxygen you can see the end of the tunnel.

[1101] Cafergot knocked the headache out in ten minutes but lost its effectiveness as the cycle wore on. Before this, nothing worked. Two years ago I had attacks so bad that I sought out a headache clinic. They saw the mental state I was in and jumped right to Prednisone. The headaches stopped.

[1102] Vigorous exercise will help reduce the pain long enough for me to go back to sleep for one-and-a-half to two hours. I tried running through the streets at two in the morning until the police asked me to stop. Now I use a rowing machine. Sometimes I row while breathing pure oxygen. When nothing else works, I use Codeine to numb the pain enough to get some sleep.

[1103] I take 100mg of Elavil at night and Fiorinal capsules. One of the best pain reliefs is to suck on ice cubes or use Ambesol to numb the area.

[1108] I have been on Eskalith, Fiorinal, Imitrex, Inderal, Toprol, Cafergot, Methysergide, and other drugs. All have worked for a short time, but have caused rebound headaches and have bad side effects. Caffeine can be effective in treating clusters. Drinking a can of Coke at the first sign of a headache works well, especially if you drink the Cola on an empty stomach. I have cans of soda with me all the time, including by my bedside. If the headache starts to come on before the caffeine kicks in I put pressure on the artery in my neck to relieve some of the pain.

[1109] I just completed a 15 day declining dosage of Prednisone. I was also taking Elavil at night before bedtime. The frequency of attacks hasn't changed, but the severity diminished. Caffeine also seems to be helpful. In the true "cluster spirit," I'll try almost anything. I have a deep breathing technique that has been successful 85 percent of the time. It can limit each attack to 20 minutes. Start immediately at the onset of a cluster. Inhale with your diaphragm, fill the lungs, hold for a few seconds, then slowly exhale, pushing with a grunting like action, first with the upper lungs, then with the lower diaphragm. It seems to stop the attack before it ever peaks.

[1110] Imitrex was a godsend for me while it worked. I had total pain relief within ten minutes. Unfortunately it stopped working.

[1111] My doctor started me on Cafergot, then switched me to Ergostat. Each worked great the first time, but not on later clusters. Then he put me on oxygen at 15 liters per minute for 15 minutes at the onset, and the pain rapidly diminished. After about five sessions they were gone! Now, four years later, they're back. I'm using Periactin, a caffeine kicker, and oxygen. Right now, oxygen seems to be the best thing for me. It helps to diminish the pain.

[1112] My husband has been given every medication used for the treatment of clusters, with very little help: Indocin, Elavil, Sansert, Verapamil, Sumatriptan, Lidocaine, oxygen, and lots more. He had a few days of relief last spring when he was given Prednisone, but it is now ineffective. In the fall he was given Carbamazepine which landed him in the hospital with serious liver complications.

[1113] I have been taking Depakote for two weeks and have not had a serious headache since.

[1116] My husband has tried everything under the sun. After three weeks of continual headaches, and many bouts to the emergency room, he was put on Lithium carbonate 900mg daily, which immediately stopped his cluster cycle. He also takes Imitrex shots, but if he takes too many, he gets rebound headaches. He tried Lidocaine, but had no response.

[1118] I've tried many different treatments. I was hospitalized for a week and put on a strong dose of steroids to break a bad cluster cycle. It did work, but I became testy and put on some weight. You can only take them for a limited time. Afterwards, I was able to control my clusters with Amitriptyline and Isoptin.

[1120] I was put on Carbamazepine during my last attack. It's most commonly given to epilepsy patients. It helped me until I developed an allergy to it. I was told that there are similar drugs, so when I need medication again, my allergy shouldn't be a problem.

[1122-F] The doctor put me on a calcium blocker that I took daily. I experienced no further headaches for one year. I stopped taking the medication and continued headache-free for several years after.

[1123] I have been on all the standard medications and am now using DHE at the onset of a headache.

[1124] I was able to stop a cluster by emptying my stomach in the bathroom. Usually my clusters last for three hours but this time it went away ten minutes after tossing my dinner.

[1131] I tried Prednisone, but have been treating my clusters with Lithium. I started with three 300mg doses a day. The headaches resumed so my doctor increased me to four pills a day. That was successful for a month, then the headaches returned. I am currently taking 1500mg of Lithium a day.

[1132] Chiropractors can't do anything. When the "warning" starts to come, a hot wash cloth usually helps. If I catch it early enough, the pain only lasts a few minutes. If I wait more than six or seven minutes to apply the compresses, then it's too late. The doctor put me on Ercaf. I take it two hours before bed and the episodes at night nearly stopped!

[1133] Two things greatly reduced my headaches: 1) Taking a daily multivitamin. This takes two to three weeks to kick in, but does reduce pain levels. 2) I stopped ingesting caffeinated food and drink — except during a headache. During a headache, a can of Coke or Pepsi actually gets rid of the headache in 20 to 30 minutes.

[1135] I gave acupuncture a chance but the clusters hurt like hell. I ended up screaming to get the needles out of my head! Oxygen was terrific for fast relief, but the pain returned very quickly, and each time it hurt a little worse than before. I now use it to hang on during the time it takes for the pain medicine to begin working.

[1138] Depakote (anti-seizure medication) bought me one season.

[1139] Vicodin is the only prescription that seems to help. Many of the other pain killers are too strong or make me sick.

[1140] After trying every drug in the pharmacy, I was fortunate to find a doctor to write a prescription for Vicodin ES, and Dilaudid 4mg for breakthrough pain. This kept the emergency room visits to a minimum. My new doctor lowered the dose. As a result, I have had several emergency room visits. I know what it takes in the emergency room: Demerol 200mg and Vistaril 100mg. The latest to my arsenal is a drug called Sensorcaine. This is mainly used as a local anesthetic by eye doctors and dentists. I used it by drawing about 3cc from the bottle, and slowly letting it drip into my nose. Prednisone also works.

[1141] What works one year won't necessarily work the next. My last prescription was for Calan, four times a day. Shooting steam straight up my nostril seems to do some good for me. Last night I was headache-free after I got a shot of Celestone (a corticosteroid). Here's a trick I learned: There's a pressure point in the web of the hand, between the thumb and index finger. At the onset of a headache, I squeeze that spot enough to give my hand a cramp and the head pain goes away within five minutes.

[1146-F] I have tried many medications. Prednisone was great in the beginning but doesn't do the trick anymore. It would stop the cycle, but another one would return and be more intense. I now rely on Cafergot suppositories. Taking a suppository really sucks, and the first few times I became sick to my stomach and dizzy, but it gets rid of the headache in minutes.

[1147] I was helped by Lithium 300mg three to four times a day plus Prozac 20mg daily. The Lithium was ineffective by itself. I need to check my Lithium level and thyroid function. I can judge my Lithium level by the severity of my tremor.

[1149] A combination of Verapamil, Lithium, and Inderal has worked for me for two months now.

[1153] My salvation has been coffee and Capsaicin. Drinking a generous amount of coffee at onset works better than any treatment I've tried.

[1156] Prednisone only helps when I am up to 60mg, which you can only take for five days. As soon as I went down to 50mg, I was back in pain. The Prednisone did shorten my cycle and buy me relief for a week or two, but it is not the cure. It makes me hyper and keeps me awake. Boy do you crash when it is all over.

[1158-F] After a year of trying to get a doctor to prescribe oxygen, I finally have something that works! I still suffer from clusters but I now have a way to fight them. At the first sign, I turn on my oxygen to 6 liters, sit on the floor in from of my recliner, put the mask on, relax, then breathe slowly and deeply. Within three minutes I feel great.

[1159] My doctor prescribed Prednisone for me, and within two days my cluster was over. A year and a half later I started another cycle of clusters. I took Prednisone again, along with Wygraine, and that worked for three days, after which the clusters returned with a vengeance.

[1160] My neurologist prescribed Prednisone 60mg for four days, 40mg for four days, and 20mg for four days. The important thing is to shut down the cycle. If there is a breakthrough headache, I use Imitrex shots (my legs are pin cushions). If the breakthroughs become more serious, I may jack up the Prednisone doses to 80mg. However, Prednisone is really bad, so I try not to do this too often. Oxygen works if you catch the headache in the beginning, but once it is going full force, it doesn't work.

[1161] Once, I had a bad attack on the road so I had my wife drive. I discovered that hanging my head out the window in 30 degree air at 60 mph provided me with the best "ice bag and fresh air treatment" I have ever had. I went out in the snow this past weekend. It was 25 degrees and the wind was blowing. I breathed slowly and deeply; within five minutes my cluster was gone. I have been on a lot of medication and seen a lot of doctors. I have been to several neurologists and to headache clinics. The only thing that has ever worked with some consistency is oxygen. It doesn't work all the time, but even if it doesn't stop the cluster completely, it seems to lessen the pain and calm me. If the oxygen doesn't help, I go to the emergency room for 100mg of Demerol. My usual drill at the hospital is for them to stick me with Demerol and leave me sucking oxygen. Then down I go for about 12 hours. However, during one episode, even the Demerol didn't help. It knocked me out after 10 minutes, but 40 minutes following the shot, another headache woke me from a dead sleep.

[1166] I take Verapamil daily during my cluster episodes, and it has worked well for me for over eight years now. After two months of taking this medication, its best to stop until the next episode comes along. I'm leery of Imitrex. I've read horror stories about side effects and seizures. Neurologists are quick to recommend it because its the hot new drug on the market and it is very expensive. I've been trying natural herbs and vitamins. I've been taking 500mg of Feverfew, and 800iu of vitamin E daily.

[1168] I've had success preventing cluster headaches by extending my day length with full-spectrum light. I also find that focusing my thoughts away from the pain can bring moments of relief.

[1169] I have tried a number of medications including Sansert, Depakote, and Prednisone. Lithium and oxygen used to be effective, but this year they do not work, and I have suffered through many episodes. I tried an Imitrex tablet. It gave me relief, but then I found out what it does. It's scary. It slows down the flow of blood through the carotid artery to your brain and can have detrimental effects on the heart.

[1170] Red pepper can be used inside the nostrils and on the nose.

[1171] I've been using oxygen for many years, and it works better than anything I have ever found. I know that as soon as I start breathing pure oxygen the pain isn't going to get any worse, and it is usually gone within 15 minutes. Keep a constant sleep cycle and stay in good physical shape. Cardiovascular exercise is good. I have noticed that the frequency and duration of clusters decreased when I ran on a regular basis. Stress is also good. When you feel a cluster coming start a task that requires your full attention.

[1174] I was a chronic sufferer but started taking 30mg of Elavil and 3mg of melatonin, and right now I am so grateful for this break that I thank God every morning. Ergotamine can subdue a cluster if taken at the first sign of an attack. Injections of Dihydroergotamine (DHE), a form of Ergotamine, are sometimes used to treat clusters. Some cluster patients can prevent attacks by taking Inderal or Methysergide. A mild solutions of cocaine hydrochloride applied inside the nose can quickly stop cluster headaches. This treatment may work because it blocks pain impulses and it constricts blood vessels. Oxygen works for some patients. In chronic cases, certain facial nerves may be surgically cut or destroyed to provide relief. These procedures have had limited success. Some cluster patients have had facial nerves cut only to have them regenerate years later.

[1177-F] I have tried everything old and new. Elavil 25mg taken at bedtime has been my only salvation for four years. I have not had a cluster during that time. I recently stopped taking it and the clusters are returning.

[1181] At the onset of a cluster headache, I jump to the floor and begin doing pushups. Anything to increase my heart rate will help.

[1183] I have managed to keep things more or less under control in recent years with a combination of Verapamil and oxygen.

[1184] I learned transcendental meditation, and my desire for alcohol, cigarettes, and marijuana diminished. My stress level dropped and now I don't suffer from clusters anymore.

[1187-F] Imitrex injections work, but the pills don't. The main thing I do to get through the pain is go to a quiet room, take a hot bath, and give myself hot compresses. This routine is mostly used for middle-of-the-night headaches.

[1189-F] Indocin works for the ice pick headaches.

[1190] Oxygen usually works. When it doesn't, my nighttime episodes respond in 30 minutes to ice packs on my cheekbone.

[1191] Imitrex pills do not work at all. I haven't tried the shot. Prednisone and Sansert usually prevent cluster headaches from occurring but some do slip through. I haven't found a drug or treatment to counter an attack once it begins.

[1193] Three weeks into my last cluster, I was prescribed Indocin. The day that I started taking it, the cluster went away. Nothing seems to work on a regular basis, although ten to fifteen minutes of oxygen will usually get rid of my clusters.

[1197] Oxygen is the fastest and cheapest way to make clusters go away. If you feel one coming on, get as much oxygen as fast as possible and the pain should subside within ten minutes. Cafergot worked a bit but made the pain worse later on. Stay off caffeine and nicotine. I tried melatonin. I knew that it could remove jet lag and resynchronize sleep patterns. Could it stabilize serotonin? I took 3mg of melatonin at 9:30 in the evening and felt good and tired an hour later. I hadn't felt like that for a long time. I slept very deeply that night and had wonderful dreams. I woke up the next morning feeling like a new person. I think it broke the cluster cycle. To resynchronize your sleep cycle, I also recommend that you turn off as many lights as possible.

[1199] I sometimes gain relief by drinking two cups of coffee, followed by a hot bath where I let my head float in the water with no pressure on my neck.

[1200] My last cluster bout was aborted with 240mg Verapamil plus Lithium. I don't know if the Lithium helped. More recently, I stopped the clusters with a double dosage of Prozac. My clusters stopped after my seventh acupuncture session, but the cluster "season" generally ends after about six or seven weeks anyway.

[1201] When my clusters get really bad, my neurologist injects Novacaine into the occipital nerve in the back of my head. This may sound bad, but for anyone who has experienced the pain of clusters, it's a walk in the park. She believes that deadening this nerve helps break the cycle. She also puts me on Inderal and Toprol during the day, and Elavil in the evening. This treatment has given me back my life.

[1203] I can relieve some of the pressure in my eye, and avert a cluster headache, by having a bowel movement. Oxygen helped, and so did Prednisone, but I don't like drugs, especially this one because it breaks down my immune system. Cluster sufferers may be ingesting pesticides that damage the hypothalamus. My clusters left once I stopped eating out, bought organic food, and went on a hypoglycemic diet. The idea is to stabilize your adrenal glands; they need a break. If pesticides or hypoglycemia are the cause of your cluster headaches, they should begin to subside and disappear within a few days to a week or so — once your body begins to readjust, and chemical regulation begins to occur. My clusters are gone. Of course, I may have been nearing the end of my cluster period. But this time I noticed a correlation between the actions that I took and their presumed effect on my clusters.

[1205-F] I take 50mg of Tenormin daily to prevent clusters, then have Darvocet on hand to use at the onset of the few remaining ones I get. I also have Imitrex for the really bad ones that hit me in the middle of the night.

[1206] Prednisone brought an immediate end to the painful monster in my head. I did suffer from diarrhea for a few days from the medication, but as I tapered off, my stomach returned to normal.

[1208] I experience some relief from milder attacks by breathing oxygen for 20 to 30 minutes. I started taking Imitrex, and I did not experience a headache for several hours. My doctor said that I should take the Imitrix with caffeine, to increase the absorption.

[1209] I have tried many medications such as Cafergot and Sansert. The only thing that works for me is Verapamil and Indocin.

[1210] Elavil has been quite effective for controlling the pain of chronic clusters despite the constant drowsiness.

[1211-F] I have tried alternative therapies such as biofeedback, relaxation techniques, Feverfew, and just about anything else you can name, without success. Now I take Tylenol #3 or Vicodin.

[1212] Elavil helped terminate my recent cluster episode in 16 days. It worked on a previous episode in ten days. Prevention depends on recognizing early signals and applying pressure to facial nerves in various ways. Aborting an attack, which I can even do when awakening to a full-blown attack, requires breathing steam from a moist heating pad called a hydrocollator which is boiled in water and wrapped in a towel. This is the only effective relief for cluster attacks that I've found. Sometimes it relieves the pain, and sometimes it actually stops the cluster within ten or fifteen minutes.

[1213] I can sometimes avoid an attack by inhaling pure oxygen. However, if the progression has gone too far, I also take 1000mg of Motrin. If the pain has still not been alleviated, I will now take a 30mg tab of Fiorinal with codeine. I can diminish some of those highly intense peaks by performing a scuba diving maneuver. This is done by holding your nose closed with your fingers while trying to blow out air. Your ears will plug up, and you may hear a squealing in your ears. This is natural, and that squeal is just air coming out of the eustachian tubes. Holding my breath and pressing on my stomach with my diaphragm will also get some results. This is like trying to make your face red when you were a kid. I also take 10mg tabs of Deltasone and 150mg tabs (twice daily) of Zantac.

[1216] I am using Lithium with Imitrex. If I don't catch it in time, the Imitrex doesn't help. A hot shower and hot air from a blow dryer, directed at my eye, mask the pain during a cluster peak.

[1218-F] Imitrex tabs work great if I catch the headache early.

[1221-F] Prednisone worked so well for me that I thought I had found my cure. But it is not good to stay on the drug very long, and every time I tapered off, I got much worse. I also puffed up and grew fine facial hair. I am a woman.

[1222] Oxygen did some good for two cycles but no longer works. Sometimes I stand over the air conditioning vent with the air on high. Showers did some good when I was younger. Prednisone did away with my headaches within three days and cut about a month off my cycle. I was still getting the puffy red eye and runny nose, and I gained 20 pounds, but was getting sleep without pain.

[1223] I tried Prednisone, Verapamil, Sansert, Lithium, oxygen, and other drugs without much success. I found some relief for a while using Lidocaine sprayed up my nostril. I am now using Cafergot, DHE-45 injections, and Nifedipine pills. When it gets really bad I'm off to the emergency room for Demerol.

[1226] I couldn't live like this anymore so I finally went to a sleep clinic. They discovered that while I slept, I would stop breathing for 30 to 45 seconds then fight for air. I'm on a breathing machine now and I have never felt so good in my life. No more headaches, Prednisone, Sansert, Lithium, or Verapamil. I am completely drug free. I feel 20 years younger, and am no longer struggling to stay awake during the day. Cluster sufferers should seriously consider checking into a sleep clinic for relief from this unbearable pain.

[1228-F] I have been on beta-blockers, Lithium, Zoloft, and much more. Suicide was prevented by the use of Cafergot, Tylenol #3, and oxygen. Oxygen at 10 liters for 20 minutes often stops the pain as fast or faster than medication.

[1229] I've been delivered from clusters twice with a combination of Prednisone, Prozac, and a strong analgesic. It's the Prednisone and Prozac that stops them.

[1234] The only thing that relieves the pain is Ergotamine tartrate — Cafergot. I tried staying off of caffeine and taking steroids, but it just doesn't work. Cold water directly on my face helps. So does extending my right arm to block the flow of blood. Total darkness is a must. My next step is to try those adhesive strips over the nose to aide breathing during sleep, because my girlfriend complains that I stop breathing at times.

[1236] When I changed to a hypoglycemic diet, my headaches went from one a week to a few every year (when I went off my diet). I am now getting relief by taking a Calcium channel blocker. As soon as I realize a headache is coming, I take up to six Midrin.

[1241] I have had good results reducing the severity of the more debilitating clusters with the herb Feverfew and cayenne peppers.

[1242] Pain can be relieved by inhaling 100 percent oxygen for 10 to 15 minutes at the beginning of the episode. Inhaling cold room air cooled to 42 degrees Fahrenheit via an inhalation device is also effective for aborting cluster headaches. Cold air and 100 percent oxygen provide equivalent pain relief.

[1243] I use very hot water in the sink or tub as a "diversion" treatment for my clusters. I put my head in the steam or under a wet towel that I heated in the microwave.

[1249] Prednisone and Fiorinal work for me, except toward the end of the bout when the headaches get really bad. I've been on 20mg of Prednisone a day for about six weeks. My doctor told me to taper the dose, but each time I do the headaches return.

[1250] I tried almost everything, including Sansert, Demerol, Percodan, and other drugs. Then I heard about someone who had used vitamin B in massive doses. I did this for three months and the headaches quit. I haven't had one in seven years now. What did it? I don't know for sure, but I'm glad they are gone.

[1251] Midrin worked for a time, but only when taken immediately upon the first twinge of pain. For the last two years Sansert has been by my side. It takes a few days to kick in (and then out again). It does have side effects and can only be used for a limited time.

[1252-F] I take two Percocet 325mg at the onset and two every two hours until it goes away. I am afraid the docs are going to cut me off soon and try to "cure" me with some exotic drugs. They ought to know that people who attempt suicide with pills need more than a few Percocet. I find that crushing the tablets and mixing with water helps it to act faster. I have tried Darvon and Stadol, which only take the edge off. I bought some Feverfew caps as a prophylactic. Codeine 3's work but make me sick. I was afraid of side effects from Ergotamine and Imitrex, but I tried Imitrex injectables at the onset and all symptoms were gone in five minutes. Except for the cost — $40 a hit and HMOs won't cover it — it seems too good to be true. My bedtime headache is still problematic, even if I try to preempt it by taking the Imitrex before its usual arrival time.

[1256] None of the usual medications — Ergotamine, Tegretol, Desyrel — gave me any relief from the pain. A high dose of Inderal stopped it within 48 hours. Tenormin is a better alternative because it has minimal side effects.

[1257] I'm using 2mg Sansert two to three times daily. This works, but can only be used for short periods of time due to side-effects, like kidney fibroma. I use Imitrex injectables when I'm off Sansert.

[1259-F] Percs stop the pain for about one-and-a-half hours. I don't know what is worse, the pain or Percocet every two hours.

[1261] A 2mg tablet of Valium will stop a headache within five minutes, or within two minutes if I chew the tablet. Two doctors I told had never heard of Valium being used for this purpose, but it works. With the combination of Valium and stretching exercises to control the buildup of tension, I have not had a full blown headache for over ten years.

[1262] In some of my worst cluster episodes I took up to eight Imitrex injections per day with no ill effects that I am aware of, although that amount is not recommended. The usual staying power of Imitrex is about four hours, although when my clusters get really bad it can come down to one-and-a-half to two hours. It was a life saver for me when I was having six to eight headaches a day. Of course, at $40 a shot, it was very expensive, but still beats the hell out of these headaches. Another drug that I just switched to is DHE. It is an injectable with less potential for cardiac problems. It is much less expensive — about $6 a shot — and works in minutes.

[1263-F] I took Toradol for a week without success. Imitrex eased the pain by about 60 percent, however the pain returned and I've had a headache almost continuously since then.

Additional Comments

In this chapter, comments are grouped into four categories: 1) About doctors; 2) Genetic and lifestyle factors; 3) Compassion and hope; and 4) Miscellaneous remarks.

About Doctors:

Cluster sufferers rely on doctors to relieve their pain, yet many complain that very few even know what a cluster headache is, their efforts are generally ineffective, and they often lack compassion.

[1069] Go to a doctor who knows what a cluster headache is.

[1086] My regular doctor was reticent to admit that a chiropractor could have correctly identified my problem.

[1087] I had no success from the many doctors I have seen.

[1101] Anyone who gets clusters should seek a headache specialist. Other doctors don't offer the time and compassion a headache specialist can provide.

[1121] My doctor does not agree with my allergy specialist, and has indicated he will refuse to work with me if I go down this road.

[1133] My doctors tell me to "just live with it."

[1140] Doctors think I'm a dope addict. They call it "drug seeking behavior." When I'm in this severe pain, and banging my head through walls, yes, I am seeking drugs. I know what works and I don't appreciate their song and dance. I have a legitimate problem. They all have access to my records, yet are reluctant to give me the shot. I needed a shot last week and the damn doctor made me wait three hours before he went for it. I've been to the pain centers, used biofeedback, and avoid triggers. But these people must go.

[1145-F] A lot of so-called experts don't seem to be knowledgeable about clusters.

[1155] Why are some doctors still unaware of cluster headaches? People are suffering and being treated for lots of other things. That happened to me. He took my money, and I suffered, because he didn't have time to read a journal.

[1157] Cluster headache treatment is a classic example of why we refer to doctors as "practicing" physicians!

[1166] My neurologist got angry with me because I kept "bothering" him. My headaches were killing me and he wants to know what I want him to do. Stop the frigging things from killing me!

[1167] I see doctors for other matters. At the typical question, "Do you suffer from any other illness?" I explain that I suffer from cluster headaches. They don't know what I'm talking about.

[1186] I'm a businessman with a family, responsibilities, yet some of these doctors treat you like a bum off the street. All of them that I've seen over the years haven't been worth five cents. I'm sorry to sound cynical, but I'm really hurting and frustrated.

[1193] I think that the term 'cluster migraine' came from doctors that don't know what the hell they are talking about.

[1194] I'm tired of doctors not knowing what this disease is about. Maybe if doctors saw photos of cluster sufferers, more research will be done and a cure might be found.

[1201] I had given up on doctors over ten years ago, but when I nearly took a gun to my head, I ventured back out to the medical world to seek help.

[1204] Heaven help us all...medical science hasn't been able to.

[1213] The first step in getting relief is finding a doctor who actually knows what a cluster is.

[1229-F] None of the doctors in my area will prescribe narcotics for my clusters. Their calling is to relieve pain and suffering, so I have a problem with that.

[1241] Don't shoot your doctor. He or she means well but probably just doesn't understand.

[1252-F] My mornings are spent in doctors' waiting rooms, and evenings under sedation. The medical establishment errs on the side of letting people suffer because they are afraid we might take a little too much and get a buzz. As a result, I have considered just buying drugs on the street. Over the weekend I ran low and had to go to a walk-in clinic to get my prescription. I had to wait an hour, then describe my symptoms and listen to a lecture about how I shouldn't just treat the symptoms but the "cause."

[1257] I've had a PA deny me a referral and had to show up at the emergency room in full-blown cluster to get their attention.

[1262] Typically, doctors are unfamiliar with cluster headaches and don't have the broad experience with the variety of medications that work for some people with clusters but not for others.

Genetic and Lifestyle Factors:

A link between cluster headaches and hereditary or lifestyle factors cannot be established due to insufficient data.

[1063] I am not overweight, I don't smoke, or snore.

[1087] My father committed suicide about 30 years ago. I strongly believe it had to do with the headaches he was known to suffer from, which I believe were clusters.

[1093] I smoke less than one pack a day and seldom drink. I do, however, drink a lot of coffee — more than ten cups per day.

[1104] I think they are hereditary. My dad got them and my brother still does.

[1106] My father is a beer drinker, smoker, and likes his caffeine.

[1145-F] I'm thin, rarely drink, and don't fit the description of the typical cluster sufferer that I've seen in literature.

[1146-F] I've been told by doctors that cluster headaches usually strike overweight men smokers in their 40s. I am a thin female.

[1156-F] I read an article that said cluster personalities are intense. My life has never been easier. I have never been more happy, relaxed, or financially secure, so I don't fit the personality features.

[1162] I've read that there is a strong correlation between body type and cluster sufferers. I am a 38 year old engineer with smooth complexion, fair skin, blue eyes, and brown hair. I am of average weight and height, don't drink or smoke, but I do eat a lot of meat and starches, and drink a lot of Coke. Because I don't seem to fit the general description, I am wondering if their data is incomplete.

[1166] My uncle had cluster headaches just like me, although nobody diagnosed them back when he had them. He had the same episodes that I now have, and at the same times of year.

[1167] I smoke, don't like alcohol, but I'm a serious Coke drinker.

[1174] The typical cluster patient is a tall, muscular man with a rugged facial appearance and a square, jutting or dimpled chin. The texture of his skin resembles an orange peel. Studies of cluster patients show that they are likely to have hazel eyes, and that they tend to be heavy smokers and drinkers.

[1184] My mother also suffered from cluster migraines, so I might have inherited them. But I firmly believe that they are caused by lifestyle.

[1219-F] I read that they are hereditary. My father also had them.

[1222] I have blue eyes and brown hair. I don't smoke or drink.

[1224] I am a professional athlete. My heart, cholesterol, and blood pressure are all near perfect.

[1235-F] If anyone says that cluster headaches are not hereditary, they need to research some more. My grandmother had them, my mother has them, and I have them.

[1260] I think that I inherited them from my father. My sister also gets them, though not as bad or as frequently as me.

Compassion and Hope:

Cluster victims gain comfort when non-sufferers try to understand what they are going through, and by simply knowing that other people suffer the same ailment and that they are not alone.

[1050] Having been a cluster sufferer for so many years, I have great sympathy and compassion for other sufferers.

[1057] It is great to share experiences with other sufferers and to know that we are not alone in this type of misery.

[1081-F] I feel sorry for cluster headache victims, and for the people close to them. I have gone through cycles with my husband, and must admit how helpless I feel. I want to hide while he suffers.

[1086] I was surprised and relieved to find that other sufferers reported similar experiences. It is a relief to simply be understood and have commiseration.

[1087] When I was 17 and literally banging my head against the wall, I would have given anything to know that there were other cluster sufferers. Just the knowledge that there are others going through the same thing gives me a lot of comfort. I've also found that knowing this is happening for a divine reason is assuring.

[1095-F] It is comforting to know that I am not the only one who suffers from these "headaches from hell."

[1101] I don't like people saying it's "only a headache."

[1111] I can cope a little better knowing I'm not alone.

[1128] It is frustrating to me when non-sufferers don't understand. I told my boss, who suffers from sinus headaches, that I had to leave, and his reply was "I had a headache last night and didn't get much sleep and I'm not leaving." Yeah, and if I only had a wimpy sinus headache for one night, I'd be there too. In fact, with only two hours of sleep in two days, and after suffering through 12 headaches of nuclear proportions, I was still at work. Another co-worker told me to just take a sleeping pill. If only they understood! Do they honestly think that when these headaches occur that I am sitting around reading a book or watching TV until it's over?

[1129-F] There is a special need on the part of the spouse for understanding. When my wife experiences the clusters, I have to become a nurse, keeper, watcher, and someone who knows when to simply go away. These things can destroy a marriage if the spouse does not understand what is needed, and sometimes to understand that absolutely nothing can be done. The person with a cluster headache becomes someone entirely different from the person you married. It is vital to the health of the marriage for the two to talk about the experience. I generally know before she does when a headache is coming. We can then plan how to approach the next several hours, and sometimes days.

[1145-F] It's so comforting to connect with others in this same miserable situation. Clusters are too awful to go it alone.

[1146-F] Good luck to fellow sufferers.

[1151] It helps me to know there are others who understand the pain I experience when I am having my episodes of torture. I used to feel that I was being punished for past wrongs, but now realize that I am not alone.

[1153] Sometimes, when I am at my lowest during an episode, I think that my suffering is meant to keep me humble and in touch with the suffering that is going on throughout the world.

[1155] It has helped me to know that I am not the only "freak" who suffers from cluster headaches.

[1161] I hate it most when people treat me like an idiot. Don't say things like "A headache? Did you take an aspirin?"

[1162] I like to know that I am not alone with the terrible "cluster monster." I wish no one had to deal with this awful problem. I offer my sincere hope that other cluster sufferers will find relief.

[1168] It's very moving to hear from other people that suffer the same as I do. I have always felt so alone.

[1171] It is frustrating to have people say "Oh yea, I used to get migraines." They have no idea of what we go through.

[1193] Everyone that I have ever tried to explain my headaches to says, "Yea, I get migraines too; I know exactly what you're talking about." I sympathize with migraine sufferers; headaches hurt. But no one understands us. They should be concerned that we don't do anything drastic.

[1220] Good luck to the few, the miserable, the cluster-sufferers!

[1222] Knowing there are others coping with this monster gives me a stiffer backbone. It is a lonely condition that happens in the middle of the night. I will not wake up my wife unless it gets to the point where I can no longer take the pain.

[1234] Thank God I've got a wonderful, understanding mate.

[1249] My wife is super. When I'm having a cluster, she'll hold me while I rock back and forth and scream, trying to reassure me that it will come to an end. She also helps by doing headache research with me. I know they scare her and she feels helpless, but there's not much more she can do besides offering me love, support, and understanding during these times. I definitely appreciate every little effort she gives.

[1257] I was treated at a headache clinic, and just being among other sufferers with shared experience made a great difference.

[1262] Anyone who describes clusters and migraines as part of a continuum doesn't understand.

Miscellaneous Remarks:

[1052] I have heard that you eventually outgrow them, but I don't know when this is supposed to occur.

[1081] Here we are in the 1990s with no more answers for cluster sufferers than they had to offer 20 years ago.

[1148] To all new cluster sufferers: You are in danger of killing yourself. Seek the attention of a competent neurologist who knows headaches. Then reflect back on what your life was like, because it just took a turn for the worse. Don't screw around...get treatment.

[1156] In Germany, seasonal headaches like clusters are referred to as "weather sickness."

[1161] Insurance pays for most of my care.

[1162] I have tried several times to keep a journal of my cluster episodes, but I am unable to keep an accurate log for some reason. This is very odd since I keep excellent records for every other aspect of my life and job. It's almost as though at a subconscious level I really don't want to remember anything about each episode.

[1164] I believe adenosine is responsible both for the dilation of blood vessels in the head and neck, and for much of the pain.

[1169] Another guy I work with also has clusters, and we both started getting them at the same time this year.

[1171] Heavy exercise will cause one side of my face to get red and flushed like it should. The other side — the side of the clusters — is ghost white. The effect is very dramatic. The line down my face is perfectly straight, from my forehead down the bridge of my nose to my adams apple. Everything on the right side is white and on the left red. I have noticed that the more frequent the clusters come the less effort it takes to produce the red/white effect.

[1174] Thermograms of untreated cluster patients show a "cold spot" of reduced blood flow above the eye. I must "crack" my neck before, during, and after a cluster attack.

[1194] Few people know about clusters except for the sufferers and their families. I've heard that about one in 10,000 have it.

[1197] Cluster headaches have been proven to subside and not be re-triggerable again for some time — a relapse period. This is similar to an epileptic seizure. I assume this is brain damage, or a malfunction of some chemical processes.

[1212] Experiencing several cluster attacks essentially unmediated by pain relievers was enlightening. Sometimes we should carefully perceive what we're trying to avoid. I could clearly differentiate between the histamine-related symptoms usually prevented by my medication (eye pain, tears, nasal congestion on one side) from the adrenalin-related symptoms (hot flashes, panic attack, and vascular spasms), which cause so much pain that they block awareness of the histamine-related symptoms when both are present.

[1222] I do not think about cluster headaches until I start having them. When this happens I can look back at the preceding week and see that I have been having symptoms. I just will not let myself think about cluster headaches until I start the cycle. I can't wait until I am finally old enough for the clusters to end. That will be the best thing about getting old.

[1229-F] I pray that God will watch over our souls, because Satan surely has our heads.

[1252-F] Before the onset of my recent cluster, I thought I had developed allergies with cold-like symptoms, except that they only lasted a couple of days.

[1257] I talk to this "thing" that coexists with me and shares my mortal being.

[1263-F] I don't want to take major medicine for life and I don't want this much pain for life either. I want to feel better and be a teen again. Please help me; I want this pain to go away. Help!

Summary and Conclusion

Cluster headaches are painful and debilitating. Victims of this awful ailment should be comforted to know that they are not alone, not forgotten, and that research is being conducted on their behalf. Cluster sufferers also have good reason to remain optimistic. The candid observations in this guidebook revealed common triggers to avoid, and opportunities to gain relief are better today than ever before. Several promising cluster treatments now exist. These were presented in the preceding pages.

Once again, good luck in your quest for a happy, healthy, and pain-free future.

APPENDIX

I. ONSET and DURATION:

Total number of cluster headache respondents in this study: 133
Gender distribution: 84% male / 16% female

A. "Current Age" Distribution Data

Average age of all respondents: 39 years old
Average age of male respondents: 40 years old
Average age of female respondents: 36 years old
Age range of all respondents: 18 to 69 years old

Under 20 years old:	3%
20 to 29 years old:	10%
30 to 39 years old:	39%
40 to 49 years old:	33%
50 to 59 years old:	11%
Over 59 years old:	4%

B. "Age at Onset" Distribution Data

Average age at onset of symptoms: 22 years old
Average age of males at onset: 23 years old
Average age of females at onset: 18 years old
Age range at onset of all respondents: 8 to 48 years old

Under 20 years old:	47%
20 to 29 years old:	37%
30 to 39 years old:	12%
Over 39 years old:	4%

C. "Duration of Ailment" Distribution Data

Average duration: 15 years (equal among male and female)
Duration range: 2 to 42 years

0 to 5 years:	14%
6 to 10 years:	20%
11 to 15 years:	21%
16 to 20 years:	23%
21 to 25 years:	13%
More than 25 years:	9%

II. RECURRING CYCLES:

Total number of cluster headache respondents in this study: 107

A. Duration Between Episodes

Average length of time between cluster episodes: 22 months

Duration range (excluding chronic cases): Some respondents reported that remission periods barely lasted two to three months; others reported that episodes came in four or five year intervals.

35% of all respondents consider their condition chronic.

54% of all respondents average at least one cluster episode annually or consider their condition chronic.

Typical responses: Episodes occur annually; every 12 to 18 months; about every 18 months; every two years.

B. Length of Episodes

Average length of each cluster episode: 10 weeks

Range: Episodes last from two weeks, to six months or longer

44% of all respondents, including chronic cases, suffer episodes averaging longer than three months.

83% of all non-chronic respondents experience episodes averaging three months or less.

Typical response: Episodes last from two to three months.

C. Daily Frequency

Average daily frequency of cluster attacks: 3 per day

Range: One every other day, to ten or more daily.

Typical responses: Attacks occur daily; one-and-a-half to two hours after falling asleep; several times a day.

D. Duration of Individual Attacks

Average duration of each cluster attack: 2 hours, 12 minutes

Range: 30 minutes to 8 hours

Typical response: Attacks last from one-and-a-half to three hours.

E. Seasonal Factors

Several respondents noted that their cluster episodes tend to occur during certain seasons. Thirty-five percent reported that they happen in the fall, 35 percent in the winter, 27 percent in the spring, and only 3 percent during the summer months.

III. TRIGGERS:

Total number of cluster headache respondents in this study: 82

A. Top Ten Most Commonly Reported Triggers

1. Alcohol
2. Smoking
3. Relaxation
4. Seasonal Factors
5. Weather Variations
6. Physiological Imbalances
7. Allergies
8. Food
9. Odors
10. Physical Trauma

Note: Although several cluster sufferers felt that stress was likely to precipitate an attack, other sufferers were equally certain that stress was not a factor. Also, several victims were able to differentiate between a cluster attack and a caffeine headache. They were convinced that caffeine is not a cluster trigger.

IV. TREATMENT and RELIEF:

Total number of cluster headache respondents in this study: 182
Total number of treatments tried: 73

A. Top Ten Most Frequently Used Treatments
(without regard to effectiveness)

1. Imitrex* 33%
2. Oxygen 30%
3. Cafergot 20%
4. Prednisone 19%
5. Verapamil 15%
6. Sansert 10%
7. Lithium 9%
8. Elavil 8%
9. Hot Shower 7%
10. Fiorinal 6%

Figures represent the percentage of respondents who tried the treatment.

B. Top Ten Most Effective Treatments
(with at least 7 respondents who tried the treatment)

1. Imitrex*   67%
2. Oxygen   62%
3. Elavil   47%
4. Caffeine   38%
5. Prednisone 37%
6. Demerol   33%
7. Inderal   29%
8. Vicodin   29%
9. Lithium   24%
10. Verapamil 22%

Figures represent the percentage of respondents
who reported that the treatment was effective
(of the total number who tried the treatment).

C. Top Ten Most Effective Treatments and/or Treatments that offered Partial or Temporary Relief
(with at least 10 respondents who tried the treatment)

1. Hot Shower 100%
2. Elavil   93%
3. Oxygen   89%
4. Imitrex*   88%
5. Prednisone 86%
6. Verapamil   85%
7. Cafergot   75%
8. Fiorinal   73%
9. Lithium   71%
10. Sansert   68%

Figures represent the percentage of respondents
who reported that the treatment was effective
or offered partial or temporary relief
(of the total number who tried the treatment).

D. Top Ten Most Ineffective Treatments
(with at least 7 respondents who tried the treatment)

1. Biofeedback 71%
2. Sansert 32%
3. Lithium 29%
4. Fiorinal 27%
5. Cafergot 25%
6. Demerol 22%
7. Verapamil 15%
8. Prednisone 14%
9. Inderal 14%
10. Imitrex* 12%

Figures represent the percentage of respondents who reported that the treatment was ineffective (of the total number who tried the treatment).

E. Type of Drug Treatments: Effectiveness
(with at least 10 respondents who tried the type of treatment)

Type	Examples	Effectiveness
Anti-Migraine	Imitrex*	67%
Oxygen	100% Oxygen	62%
Anti-Depressant	Prozac, Elavil, Desyrel, Imipramine, Zoloft	50%
Steroid	Prednisone	37%
Vasoconstrictor	Caffeine, Cafergot	22%
Channel Blocker	Verapamil	22%
Beta-Blocker	Inderal, Tenormin, Toprol	20%
Anti-Convulsant/ Sedative	Valium, Depakote, Tegretol, Midrin	19%
Narcotic Analgesic	Demerol, Darvon, Dilaudid, Percocet	18%
Misc. Drug	Sansert, Codeine, Stadol, Lidocaine, Sudafed, Wygraine	16%
Anti-Inflammatory	Aspirin, Ibuprofin, Indocin, Naprosyn, Toradol	12%
Analgesic	Aspirin, Tylenol, Midrin, Fioricet, Fiorinal, Vicodin	10%

Figures represent the percentage of respondents who reported that the treatment was effective (of the total number who tried it).

F. Alternate Names for Drugs

Common Name	Alternate Name
Cafergot	Ergotamine, Ercaf, DHE
Darvon	Darvocet
Elavil	Amitriptyline
Ibuprofin	Advil, Motrin
Imipramine	Tofranil
Imitrex	Sumatriptan
Lithium	Lithonate, Eskalith
Prednisone	Deltasone
Sansert	Methysergide
Tegretol	Carbamazepine
Toprol	Lopressor
Verapamil	Calan, Isoptin
Vicodin	Hydrocodone

Notes on Imitrex and Oxygen

*Imitrex was the most frequently used and highly rated cluster treatment. Sixty of 182 respondents had tried it at least once. Of these, 40 considered it effective, 13 said it offered some relief or temporary help, while only seven rated it ineffective.

Imitrex may be ingested or injected. Of the 12 respondents who used the Imitrex pills, six considered them effective while six rated them ineffective. Of the 14 who used the injectable form of Imitrex, 10 considered it effective while the remaining four stated that it offered some relief or temporary relief. Thirty-four other respondents used Imitrex but did not specify which form they used. Twenty-four of them rated it effective, nine thought it provided some relief or temporary relief, and one claimed it was ineffective.

Although Imitrex was highly rated, many of the respondents who tried it had serious concerns about its potentially dangerous side-effects, the high cost to acquire it, and the severe rebound headaches that seemed to coincide with increased use of this drug.

Oxygen was the second most frequently used and highly rated cluster treatment. Fifty-five of 182 respondents had tried it at least once. Of these, 34 rated it effective, 15 said it offered some relief or temporary relief, while only six rated it ineffective.

Although oxygen was frequently used and highly rated, no side-effects were reported. In addition, several respondents happily noted that it is relatively inexpensive to acquire.

INDEX

Purchasing Information

Additional copies of this book, **Cluster Headaches: Treatment and Relief** (ISBN: 1-881217-18-3), may be obtained directly from *New Atlantean Press*. Send $9.95 (in U.S. funds), plus $3.50 shipping, to:

New Atlantean Press
PO Box 9638-925
Santa Fe, NM 87504

Credit Card Orders: 505-983-1856

This book is also available at many fine bookstores.

Bookstores and Retail Buyers: Order from Baker & Taylor, Ingram, Midpoint Trade Books or from New Atlantean Press. Libraries may order from their favorite library wholesaler.

Doctors, Neurologists, Headache Specialists, and other Non-Storefront Buyers: Take a 40% discount with the purchase of 5 or more copies of this book (multiply the total cost of purchases x .60). Please add 7% ($3.50 minimum) for shipping.

Shipping: Books are usually shipped within 24 hours. Please allow one to three weeks for your order to arrive, or include $3.50 extra for priority air mail shipping. Foreign orders must include 9% ($4 minimum) for shipping; $6 each for air mail. Checks must be drawn on a U.S. bank, or send a Postal Money Order in U.S. funds. **Sales Tax:** Please add 6% for books shipped to New Mexico addresses.

FREE CATALOG: *New Atlantean Press* offers nearly 200 books and videos on cutting-edge alternative health solutions, natural immunity, progressive parenting, natural childcare, AIDS, cancer, and more. Send for a free catalog. Or visit our internet website:

http://thinktwice.com/books.htm